33 KEYS TO ASCENSION

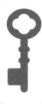

A COMPREHENSIVE GUIDE FOR ASCENSION & ENLIGHTENMENT FOR THE MODERN-DAY WORLD

channeled by Rae Chandran
with Robert Mason Pollock

**Other Books by Rae Chandran
with Robert Mason Pollock**
Angels and Ascension
Dance of the Hands
DNA of the Spirit, Volume 1
DNA of the Spirit, Volume 2
Partner with Angels

Other Books by Rae Chandran
Rumi's Songs of the Soul

33 *K*EYS
TO
*A*SCENSION

A
COMPREHENSIVE
GUIDE FOR
ASCENSION & ENLIGHTENMENT
FOR THE
MODERN-DAY WORLD

channeled by Rae Chandran
with Robert Mason Pollock

Light Technology PUBLISHING

For information about special discounts for bulk purchases, please contact Light Technology Publishing Special Sales at 1-800-450-0985 or publishing@LightTechnology.net.

ISBN-13: 978-1-62233-062-1
ebook ISBN: 978-1-62233-796-5

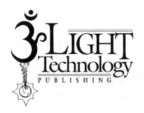

Light Technology Publishing, LLC
Phone: 1-800-450-0985
1-928-526-1345
Fax: 928-714-1132
PO Box 3540
Flagstaff, AZ 86003
LightTechnology.com

This book is for those who seek the light in all its glory — for the highest good for themselves and for others — in every moment of their lives.

Contents

ℱreface

Robert Mason Pollock

Rae Chandran and I have worked on five books together over the past five years. I feel that this book contains the most powerful material and the deepest teachings of the five. I am honored and humbled to have participated in unveiling these practices and to have been the first to learn them. These were among the most profound experiences of my life, and more than once I was brought to tears.

Rae teaches workshops throughout Asia and leads tours of sacred sites all over the world. The idea for this book came from Rae. Many of his students asked him how they could work toward ascension, so he asked and prayed for guidance. The resulting systematic practices and teachings take the seeker step by step on a pilgrimage to enlightenment.

Rae lives outside Tokyo, and I live in the United States, so all the sessions for this book were conducted over the internet on Skype. We followed this practice for the other books, and up to ten people from all over the world participated in those sessions. My role then was to record the sessions and track down the participants whose

Skype connections had dissolved, and I felt like a ringmaster who was unable to enjoy the circus. So this time, only Rae and I did the sessions along with the Family of God.

The Family of God is the combined consciousnesses of Archangel Metatron, Master Mahareya, and King Akhenaton. They worked together to organize the material in this book, and they occasionally called on others for help.

I have not ascended yet, but working with this material has given me some of the most profound experiences of my life. I have felt nonphysicality — what it is like to exist as a point of light in the cosmos. I have felt lifted into higher dimensions — less dense, as if I could walk through a wall. I have entered the vesica piscis within my heart. And I have become reacquainted with Osiris. He now lives in my heart.

You will have similar experiences. Call on your guides and the masters and archangels you work with. They will help you sustain what you experience through these practices. They are present in your life and will support your efforts when you ask.

Ascension takes work, and Earth needs enlightened residents. It will not come with a solar flash or be triggered by a celestial event. May the light be with you!

Introduction

The Family of God

Greetings to all. This book is for those who seek the light in all its glory — for the highest good for themselves and for others — in every moment of their lives. This book is for the people who say, "I want to know God within me." It is for everybody who seeks communion, a oneness, with God.

Since time immemorial, people have sought a gentle approach to connecting with the Divine and becoming the Divine. Throughout Earth's history, many have attempted to teach this to their students and others who seek the light. But there never has been a comprehensive text or material systematically outlined, step by step, in a simplified manner that a layperson could understand and practice.

This book is not written from a high place of spiritual evolution. It is written from a layperson's perspective. It shares information that all people can follow and practice. They can be what they seek. All on the path seeking higher light will find this material easy to use, for there is truth in this book. There is energy behind every word. Every meditation was shared and experienced by Robert and others. This speaks of the validity of what we are saying — the energy behind the words, the energy behind the masters.

When you are ready to embrace their light, simply open your heart and say, "I take in the energy of every word so that it becomes imprinted on my soul and the very fiber of my being. Now it opens its energy within me so that I can experience it."

The beauty of this book is that, after a few chapters, the readers will feel that they already know the answers. They will already know the next step they need to take. So in many ways, this book simply states what all of you already know within your beings. We are just mirroring back to you your innermost truth.

The Teaching Format of This Book

Many lightbeings agreed to contribute to this book, but they requested we say that all the material comes from a collective, the Family of God. The Family of God is the combined consciousness of Archangel Metatron, Master Mahareya, and King Akhenaton.

Should the format for this book be a dialogue, or should it be an exercise book? When there is a dialogue, some people are able to relate personally, and the exercises and experiences become personal tips. We have found that the experiences of a few can benefit many. If it is just a workbook, it is like any other book. But when someone experiences these energies as they are given, this can become a catalyst for others.

Some people might not feel anything initially because people have different strengths and capacities for attainment. But when they read others' experiences, they can relate. Some might feel that nothing happened to them, and they might conclude that they are not doing well or that the material is not good. Thus, from our viewpoint, it is best to have a personal dialogue. It is a humble dialogue, and it relates personal experiences of this material.

This material is comparable to the love energy that was dispersed by Master Yeshua. His energy permeated the love of God through every word he said and even when he did not speak. Jesus said that through him you can find what you seek. So the energy is the same.

Although many masters came through for this book, we would like to acknowledge the greatest teachers, Archangel Michael, who brings people together and also Mother Mary. Always remember, these two beings of light have been holding energy for the planet for millions of years. So we would like to acknowledge them in this book, for they are the overseers of the whole process.

We are the Celestial Beings of Light and the Family of God. Thank you.

Maintain the Layers of the Aura

The Family of God

Family of God: We are emissaries from the Creator, honoring the prayer and the request made by Rae to the Creator to bring forth understanding in an easy-to-understand manner so that laypeople can learn the process to help them evolve. This prayer has been answered, and we are honored to bring you this information.

We believe this information is very valuable. We have noticed that although people have a desire to ascend, they are not able to follow one clear path. They do many things at once without a clear methodology. They might do one thing today and something else tomorrow. If they were able to follow straightforward guidelines, their work would be accelerated. Otherwise, they would still reach their destination but at a much slower pace. What we wish to bring forth are clear directions that you can follow for which you can say, "I am fully ready to embrace the light, and I am going to follow this process to do so."

We refer to this book as the "keys to ascension." Keys open doors. When you open a door to ascension, you stay in that room for a while,

1

familiarize yourself with it, and then integrate the energies there. Then you go to the next room. You cannot go to the next room until you go through the first. Each step is similar. In following the steps in this book, you follow one door to the next door, and you take energy from one step to the next. The intention of this book is for you to accumulate wisdom through every step so that you will have the energy you need to make shifts within you.

This material is for dedicated students who say, "I am fully ready to commit to my path of self-liberation." This will require making a complete commitment to be on the path and do the exercises as they are given. This is very important. Only then will you be able to accelerate your growth and reach the goal of ascension, which may take three to five years, depending on your soul growth when you started the process, as well as other factors.

Aura Maintenance

Everybody has heard about the human aura. The upkeep of your aura is critical to maintaining higher frequencies of light. When there are holes in your aura, your life force seeps out. You feel drained or lethargic and generally not well mentally, emotionally, and physically. So we are taking this understanding to a higher level.

Ascension key 1 is for aura maintenance and understanding the aura. The human aura is like a sheet of very fine, thin, mist-like energy around your physical body.

Layer 1: the Pain Body (Orange Red)

The first layer of the auric field is called the pain body. It is an orange-red color. This is expanded in many human beings. It has completely overcome many people, and they carry large pain bodies. One reason people hurt each other is that they are in pain. They act out. Their pain is from either their own actions or some perceived injustice done to them.

Any time people attack others through words, thoughts, or deeds, they are expressing from their pain bodies. Pain bodies interact with each other and strongly influence your actions. Many violent people carry large pain bodies like big balloons around them.

As a lightworker, you must heal your pain body:

1. Bring light from your heart to your pain body.
2. Visualize your pain body aura as orange red, and breathe into it. See this energy surround you.
3. See yourself fully bathed in the light of your soul.

Layer 2: the Anger Body (Dark Olive Green)

The second layer of the aura is called the anger body. It is strongly connected to the pain body. Those with an anger body feel angry with themselves, their parents, society, their country, and God. Many Islamic terrorists are angry with America. When you talk with them, they will tell you, "We are not angry at the American people, but we are angry toward the ideology America holds."

People are angry for a variety of reasons. You might hear people say the following:

- "I am angry because I was born poor."
- "I didn't have the same opportunities other people had."
- "My parents left me when I was very young, so all my problems come from that."

People describe a number of sources for their anger. What they do not realize is they have choices. It does not matter what the situation was, if you feel in control, you will not feel angry. Anger toward anything — a foreign policy, a government, or an event — creates an anger body, and this body stays with you.

If the anger body is not healed, the anger will accumulate. Anger can become rage, and rage can turn into violence, such as harsh words or physical force. You must heal this body by sending it light and love.

Layer 3: the Love Body (Light Purple)

The third part of the auric energy is called the love body. The color is light purple. This is the body many masters don after their full integration, and it becomes a part of them.

Love has many forms. Love is silence. Love is acceptance. Love is forgiveness and compassion, and love is universal. Love is action. Love is sharing. Most important, love is caring.

This body needs to be active but not to the degree that you live your life only in love. Love exists in all human beings even when it is only displayed at certain moments or toward certain people. It is always present in the auric body, and you must actively seek this body and bring it forth. You must integrate it with the other bodies. All your etheric bodies spin around your physical body. Simply ask that these bodies be activated and balanced. Visualize a small gap between each body. The colors will vibrate slowly at first, and then they will vibrate faster and faster, extending to the top of your head and then falling around you like a fountain. You can ask for help from any of your etheric bodies as situations arise in your life.

Layer 4: the Ancestral Body (Pale White)

The next auric body is called the ancestral body. This is very important, but not because your coloring, hair, body type, and many other things are influenced by your genetic lineage. Many people do not understand that the ancestral body also contains traits, belief systems, sicknesses, hardships, and imprints that have been transmitted to you. You carry these traits with you, and they influence your subconscious mind. Deep down, you might believe that life is hard because your ancestors went through very hard times. Simply ask that these bodies be activated and balanced, as provided in layer 3.

Layer 5: the Compassionate, or Buddha, Body (Light Green)

The next auric body is the compassionate, or Buddha, body. True compassion means true acceptance in allowing other people to be who they are. This is what made Master Yeshua so special. When he met people, he accepted their belief systems and their ways of life, and he had only love for them. He did not say, "Your belief system, your way of understanding God, is wrong." He simply loved them for who they were.

The Dalai Lama does the same. He does not preach Tibetan Buddhism (although he may talk about it). He loves everybody, and he has compassion in his heart. This is a very important quality for ascension. Millions of lightworkers can feel energy. Some can see colors, but they aren't able to grow because there is no love, compassion, or generosity in their hearts. Compassion, generosity, and sharing must become a part of your spiritual cloth, because then you will have creativity in your life.

Layer 6: the Explorer Body (Metallic Blue and Gold)

The next layer is called the explorer body. This body is a person's ability to see the larger picture, the larger truth — the forest for the trees. It is the ability to imagine something in a larger capacity rather than defined by its individual existence. This body is activated in many young people and entrepreneurs, for they have dreams that they work toward until they reach them.

People who have gone to the North Pole or South Pole, people who have crossed great oceans, or people like Thomas Alva Edison have fully active explorer bodies. Such people do not accept life just as it seems. Instead, they strive to achieve something beyond their personal scope of life to make things much better for themselves and humanity. Simply ask that these bodies be activated and balanced, as provided in layer 3.

Layer 6-A: the Creative Body (Pale Orange)

This small body is attached to the explorer body. It is active in small children. They lie in front of the television or on the floor and draw things. They'll draw houses, their mommies, gardens, trees, flowers, or birds. Their imaginations are very active, and adults try to curb that.

Unless the creative body is opened, a person will always be stuck. They cannot grow. They start doing repetitive things because these are comfortable, but they lack a zest for life. Many people live like this. They exist without enthusiasm, and they continue in the same patterns. Simply ask that these bodies be opened and balanced, as provided in layer 3.

Layer 7: the Peace Body (Pure White)

The next auric body is the peace body. Peace simply means wisdom. Peace is a choice. Are you peaceful with yourself? Are you peaceful with your immediate family? Are you peaceful with your friends, colleagues, and neighbors? Are you peaceful with your culture and with your country? Are you peaceful with Earth? Are you at peace with God?

Layer 8: the Star Body (Silver)

The next body is called the star body. This auric energy represents the lineage of your life on other planets, star systems, and galaxies. Everyone has lived beyond Earth. You carry these imprints within you.

The star body also contains the qualities, traits, and higher frequencies you had on higher-dimensional planets when you incarnated there. It also contains the star codes, star frequencies, and star vibrations.

Layer 9: the Frequency, or Musical, Body (Magenta)

The next auric body is called the frequency, or musical, body. Human beings are very finely tuned to sound. You hear sound from the time you wake up until you go to bed. Even when you are sitting in your house, you often can hear the sound of a passing car, water dripping from the roof, or any number of other sounds.

Sound greatly affects your aura and your very being much more than is understood. Music from the radio while driving or electronic music from a CD can have a very big impact on you. What kind of music are you playing? Who composed it? What are the rhythms? What is the melody? Heavy metal and rap music [if you don't like it] can damage your aura very quickly. It could cause you to feel tired, angry, or restless.

Certain musical notes can calm your state of mind. People who work on a production line might whistle or sing, and they feel good. Children babble and sing when they are small because it makes them feel good. When you sing, your body can be nourished and uplifted.

Layer 10: the Night, or Moon, Body (Pale Indigo)

The next auric body is called the night, or moon, body. Human beings need to be nourished by the night. But modern humans rarely spend time outdoors at night or where there is no artificial light. This is almost impossible in a city. The Moon nourishes us. The Moon rules our subconscious minds and our emotions. Simply spending time under the night sky without any lights for 30 minutes to 1 hour per week is all that is needed to balance this aspect.

You will feel a sense of calmness and peacefulness because the night body properly enlarges its energy. This affects your endocrine system, kidneys, and bloodstream. It balances your thoughts, feelings, and emotions, influencing the words you use to express yourself. When you spend 2 hours sitting under the night sky — not listening to music, just being still — you can be transported to another reality. Your dreams will be very powerful, and when you awake in the morning, you will feel exuberant.

Layer 11: the Sun, or Luminous, Body (Platinum)

The next layer is called the sun body. The Sun is the giver of life. The Sun nourishes everything. Why do you think people have problems creating even when they have put much effort into trying? This is because they do not have sun energy in them. For example, when caring for a plant or a seed, you can water it, but it also needs sunshine to grow.

When there is little sun energy in the physical body, there is not much light. Sun energy simply helps you move out of darkness. When your sun body is fully activated, it is called the luminous body, and every cell vibrates with sun consciousness. This means your body is vibrating with the consciousness of the light. Simply ask that these bodies be activated and balanced, as provided in layer 3.

Layer 12: the Dream Body (Beige)

The next body is called the dream body. The dream body is where you process information and karmic energy when you sleep. Karmic energies are very dense and heavy. Your soul supports you in healing this dense karmic energy during sleep so that you do not have to bother with physical experiences. You work in your sleep to heal these karmic energies. You can program your dream body to find solutions to your everyday life conditions. Simply ask that the dream body be activated and balanced, as provided in layer 3.

Layer 13: the Wisdom, or Master's, Body (Brilliant White)

The next layer is the wisdom, or master's, body. The color is a beautiful, brilliant white. Your wisdom body contains the truth about who you are. The truth about everything is embedded in this body. When you fully awaken this body, you set yourself free. Wisdom liberates. Simply ask that these bodies be activated and balanced, as provided in layer 3.

Layer 14: the Water Body (Blue)

The last layer is called the water body. The water body represents the fluids in your physical system, including the blood, supporting the full functioning of your physical body. When the water body is fully activated and balanced, your emotional energy is well balanced. When your emotional energy is well balanced, your mind is balanced. Your mind is feminine, and when the mind is balanced, the feminine brings forth new wisdom and new light, and it births new consciousness. Simply ask that these bodies be activated and balanced, as provided in layer 3.

Integrate and Repair Your Auric Field

These bodies are part of your auric system. When you sleep, meditate, or pray, your guides bring information that flows directly from the Creator into your auric field, and it stays there. This is one reason that you cannot remember that guidance after you wake up in the morning. You might have a vision of traveling to a temple or a healing center, but when you come back, you are not able to fully remember the experience. However, it stays in your aura.

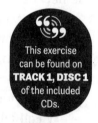

This exercise can be found on **TRACK 1, DISC 1** of the included CDs.

Sometimes your other bodies are more active, especially the pain body and the anger body, so the guidance gets numbed deep inside. When you heal these bodies and balance your auric field, you can remember more and feel healed and balanced. Your auric bodies contain your akashic record and your mind. Your mind is everywhere, but the concentrated energy of the mind is in the auric body.

1. Imagine you are sitting or standing, and there are fourteen circles surrounding you — one circle encasing the next.
2. Between each circle is a small gap. Imagine that in this small gap, there is one auric body. You might want to paint an image of this to help you visualize: fourteen colors in the fourteen circles.
3. As you breathe, see these circles vibrating. See yourself in the middle of the circles. Breathe into this image.
4. Initially, the colors vibrate slowly. Then they vibrate faster and faster.
5. You see them coming into you slowly, entering your entire body. Feel these colors within you.

6. See these colors come up through the top of your head like a fountain of light and then pour down into your aura.

Do this exercise once a day for a minimum of 21 days. This will help you repair your auric body. When you do it sincerely for 21 days, you will see a change in your thinking and your mental capacity. When you become aware of these bodies, you can tune in to a specific auric body to bring forth the energy you need at that time:

- When you are looking for wisdom or a solution to a problem, tune in to your wisdom body. Breathe into the wisdom body.
- When you're looking for peace, breathe into the peace body, and you'll be able to tap into that energy because it is a part of your auric field. It is always there with you.

Simply make the intention that you are doing this to balance, harmonize, and heal your auric body. The first step toward raising your frequency is maintaining the auric field and increasing the light of your aura. In three weeks, you will have integrated the energies within you.

When you wake up on the morning of day 22, simply say, "I awaken all my auric bodies, and I ask that all my auric bodies be completely balanced." Making that intention will activate your auric body. You manifest your intention through this. Intention is key in the new consciousness.

Retrieve and Reintegrate Soul Fragments

The Family of God

Family of God: Ascension key 2 is about soul integration — collecting soul fragments that have split from your consciousness during the many lifetimes you have had on Earth and in other realities. This is a very important task, just as aura maintenance is. You must call forth the fragmented parts of your soul and make a conscious effort to reintegrate them.

When humans are traumatized, their energy fields collapse. When the energy field collapses, there is soul fragmentation. Part of the soul leaves the body, and unless the person can get that part back, he or she will always remain in a place of nervousness, anxiety, depression, or something similar.

Soul fragmentation happens on all levels simultaneously. During a traumatic death, soul fragmentation is much more serious. For example, brother Robert, in a past life, you lived in Rome where you were a soldier. You were wounded, and you were left to die because it was burdensome to carry you back. You felt lonely, hopeless, and helpless. During the last moment of your life, you thought, "I am alone."

You felt betrayed by your comrades, the ruler, and your god. In that moment, a large part of your soul fragmented. You can call this part of your soul to the light during meditation.

Soul fragmentation happened for many people when they were persecuted for their religious beliefs. During the moment of death, their souls fragmented. They might have been expelled from a tribe or community and cast out to live alone in the world.

Almost all humanity has gone through similar circumstances. All humanity has had soul fragmentation. When Atlantis sank, many people drowned. There was incredible sadness, loss, and soul fragmentation because when the waters started rising, fear rose from the deepest levels. Imagine how many lifetimes you had and how many fragments you created.

It is said that during an average lifetime, between 1 and 5,000 soul fragmentations happen before a person reaches thirty years old. Behavior from a strict father, a demanding mother, or a stern kindergarten teacher or even a police officer can cause fragmentation. Healing these fragmentations is very important. You must bring these parts back and integrate them to feel whole and to access the talents and gifts in them.

There is a shamanic practice used by Native Americans and other people called soul retrieval. They did this for soldiers who went to war. After returning from war, many soldiers had posttraumatic stress disorder. They saw atrocities on the battlefields, and their souls could not accept such sorrow — how one human being could dehumanize another. Soul retrieval is a very effective practice.

Soul fragmentation can be done daily. You must call these parts back to you because they are part of your consciousness. They contain light and other qualities and experiences. They are part of your aura and your luminous body (layer 11), and they are important for unifying and healing your auric field. Soul fragments contain the essence of who you are.

Unifying your soul fragments is a very important part of your ascension process and can be done by simply calling the fragmented parts to return to you. There is a mudra, or hand gesture, to help you accomplish this [see figure 2.1].

Extend the fingers of your left hand. All fingers touch each other, and your left thumb rests on the index finger. Your left wrist touches

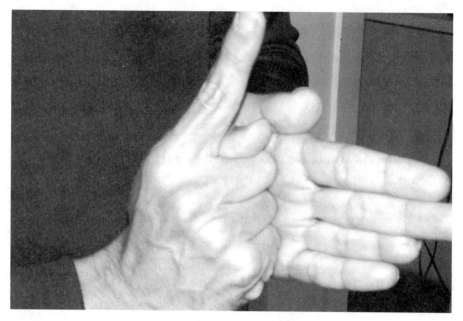

Figure 2.1. Mudra to unify your soul fragments

your solar plexus, and your fingers point away from your body. The middle, ring, and pinky fingers of the right hand rest on your right palm. Your right thumb rests on these three fingers, and your fist touches the palm of your left hand. Your right index finger points upward.

Hold your hands in this configuration in front of your solar plexus, breathe, and say, "I call forth all the lost parts of my soul to return to me at the ages I specify." Only the energy will return, not the experience or the trauma. The energies will be naturally cleansed, whole, and purified. They will return in a pretrauma state. You do not have to state this; it will happen as part of the process.

Should all the soul fragments be called back at once, or should we pace this?

When you start this practice, the lost parts of your soul will not return all at once. They will return in increments.

Nevertheless, we should ask for all?

Ask for all the parts, and your soul will regulate how much you can handle. It will become continuous. Tone the sound "shuhuei." Initially, you might feel some discomfort. You might feel some nausea and some head spinning.

I feel some of that.

There are colors of light. Try it now.

I'm doing that, and I feel the nausea.

Close your eyes, and say, "I call forth the lost parts of my soul from the Roman life."

I call forth the lost parts of my soul from a Roman life. Yes, I can feel the disorientation, the feeling of being lost and abandoned.

Now you stay there for 2 to 3 minutes, and just breathe it in. Don't be afraid. Breathe it in. Your body might feel uncomfortable.

It's settling in nicely now. When I went to a mystery school in Canada, we had a technique for integrating returning parts. We used an invocation to clear ourselves that seems similar to this. We had many parts coming back as part of this process. Is that similar to what you're saying?

There are many ways of doing things. We are bringing forth this understanding with a mudra. This is the quickest way to do it. Because of the planetary shift in consciousness, you will see this happening very quickly without needing to understand the procedure.

So we should just feel it, bring it in, let it heal, and let it integrate.

Usually, you will start feeling much better in 3 to 5 days. You will feel rejuvenated and as if something that was lost has returned. There are many ways you can approach this, and you can work out your own methodology. You are probably not going to know where each fragment was from or when it lived. You could say, "I call forth the lost parts of my soul, especially ones that I lost during traumatic death experiences in past lives." You should hold this thought for several minutes or until it feels as if it has passed.

Since you have had so many lives, this must be done for several consecutive days because fragments of your soul will return each day. If you created between 1 and 30 soul fragments per year, just imagine how many fragments are out there. It could take many days, so this should be a daily process. You could do it for several months, maybe 3 to 5 minutes a day.

This is best done before you go to sleep or during meditation. This work can be more powerful if you do it in power vortexes or other power places on Earth. The energy is much stronger there, and you will be able to call for more parts to return. That is the optimum condition.

You could choose to do this work in age increments. For example,

"I call forth soul fragments from all lifetimes before I was five years old." Then you could call for fragments from five to ten years, ten to fifteen years, fifteen to twenty years, and so forth. You could do this systematically. You decide how you want to do it, but in every lifetime, you have had many incidents during which you lost soul parts.

It's amazing how easily the human psyche is bruised by these emotions.

Exactly. This is not very well understood by the mainstream, so we encourage people on the ascension path to follow this procedure on a regular basis, and they will see huge changes. Not only will they start feeling better, but also many new talents and abilities that were in those lost parts will blossom. Your aura is strengthened by the returning energy.

Call for Your Soul Fragments to Return

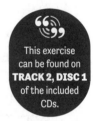

This exercise can be found on **TRACK 2, DISC 1** of the included CDs.

You can call on Master Sananda to support you in this work. He is part of Yeshua's, or Jesus's, soul, like a branch of a tree, where the branch takes on its own life. He is the master of the integration of soul fragments. There is also a goddess who works to support this integration: Hea Ma. She is a goddess in her reality, another planetary dimension, and she works with children who have had traumatic soul loss from abuse or trauma when they were born, such as being born prematurely or by cesarean section. These babies are put in little boxes and are completely separated from their mothers. There is incredible soul loss for children so tiny. They can feel betrayed by the ones who gave them life. The lights and noise of a hospital do not have sacredness. The conditions are very inhumane.

Rae had an experience when he was in Florida this year. A woman came to see him, crying. She told him that she had made a grave mistake. When her son was born, she told him, "You look so ugly." She was a very beautiful woman, and she said from that moment on, she and the child were never on good terms. He's now thirty-nine years old. He does not communicate with her or want anything to do with her. She regrets saying those harsh words as she looked into her son's eyes after he was born. Just imagine the soul loss for the child!

People like this woman's son can say, "I call forth all the lost parts of my soul, even the parts I am not aware of in this lifetime," because many people are not aware that they lost soul fragments when they were very young.

All sorts of soul loss occurred during World War II. There were destructive bombings, night raids, and loud sirens. Some people were vaporized in the bombings. Many children were terrified when they were told to hide in their basements. There was great sorrow and fear of who was going to knock on the door tonight: "Will the SS take my father away?"

You're saying that in one session, people can call for all the soul losses from one to five years old, for example, or during birth. This is going to take many months.

Many, many months. Each time you do it, you will feel stronger.

I think from what I felt when I did this that I would know from feeling whether anything is coming back, and if not, it would be time to move on to another phase.

There can be some sadness initially, but this sadness is like a mist, and it will vanish once the integration happens.

Will we be able to tell whether anything is actually happening?

Yes. You will feel it, all the past experiences. You will feel that discomfort in the body — the sadness, sorrow, and betrayal. So this is the practice. Make it a daily routine, like brushing your teeth: "I call forth all the lost parts of my soul to come back to me during the time it happened, and I call Master Sananda and Goddess Hea Ma to support me so that I can handle this energy and so that this energy becomes a part of my everyday life."

Just breathe it in. You can light a candle if you like. You can call on your guides to bring supportive energy. They will surround you with love so that you are not afraid.

1. First, set up your methodology. Age groups, births, or traumatic deaths are some examples.
2. Next, ask for help from Master Sananda, Goddess Hea Ma, and your guides.
3. Say, "I call forth the lost parts of my soul to return to me now." Specify age grouping or other methodology.
4. Make the sound "shuhuei."
5. Breathe.
6. Spend at least 3 to 5 minutes doing this, longer if you feel the process needs more time.

Heal with Sacred Temple Energy

The Family of God

Family of God: Ascension key 3 is about the many temples and places of sacred teaching and healing you can visit on the inner planes. We strongly urge you to go to these temples regularly to do the work that they are designed for. We have included images so that you can work with these temples in your meditations. You don't have to visit these temples every day. Sometimes you will work with a temple for one day or a few days, and when you release or forgive, you will know something has changed inside, and you won't have to go back right away.

The Types of Temples Available

The Temple of Love: You can visit this temple during meditation to reconnect with the energy of love. Many people are not able to feel love. Although they want to feel it, they are not able to, which means they also cannot express it. For many people, love is just a concept or a theory rather than

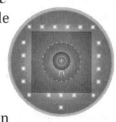

an experience. Visiting this temple can awaken understanding about all aspects of love and how to express it moment to moment.

How do you express love to a child? How do you express love to a spouse? How do you express love to a waiter in a coffee shop, a gas station attendant, or a patient whose condition is serious? The ways we treat people are how we express love, and we express love in many forms. How do you express love from your heart center to everyone? Is this the same love you extend to your children?

The Temple of Love can also purify the essence of love within you, and it can also increase the love potion within you. The pineal gland is called the love gland. When this gland is fully activated, you are able to express love almost all the time. The masters of the pineal gland help you activate it.

Despite difficulties, you will be able to express love almost all the time. Even when there is danger to life, you are capable of expressing love. We encourage people to go to the Temple of Love on the inner planes to open your hearts more fully and realize love in all its aspects.

The Temple of Sound: There is a circular door that leads into this temple. Inside there are strobe lights and a chair in the middle. You can sit on this chair, ask to bring the appropriate light frequency, and select strobes of light to fall into you. You are attuned to several sounds. Sounds can elevate you very quickly because sounds bypass your various minds — unconscious, subconscious, and superconscious — and take you directly to the source.

There are tones that must be made by the human voice. These tones resonate with you. You all have from seven to nine sounds that, when sung properly, can help you transcend to another reality.

When you go to the Temple of Sound, you can also tone your soul frequency name, and this sound will be expanded. Any sound you make in the Temple of Sound will be expanded, simply chant "Kadosh, Kadosh, Kadosh Adonai Tze'va'ot."

"Kadosh" means "holy," and this sound frequency can directly connect you to the source of life itself. When you go to the Temple of Sound, you can chant this or simply chant your name. The frequency of any chant you make in this temple will be amplified, and you will be filled with this light.

How do we know our soul frequency?

Your soul has a sound frequency embedded in a crystal where your crystals are kept, the cave of creation. This is one of the keys we will be talking about. You will visit the cave of creation regularly.

The Temple of Forgiveness: This is a temple for people who have difficulty letting go. Go to this temple and say, "I am asking to release ___." Because of the higher frequency in this temple, you will be able to let it go.

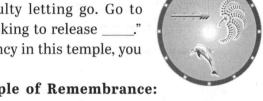

The Temple of Remembrance: We suggest that you frequent the temple of remembrance to recall who you are. Imagine you are sitting in this temple. In front of you burns the sacred flame of purification. It blazes away dense energies within you. You will be purified and remember more of who you are.

The Temple of Compassion: You can go to this temple to develop compassion and acceptance. Ask to have compassion for other human beings. You must fully integrate these qualities for ascension.

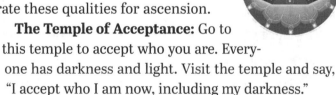

The Temple of Acceptance: Go to this temple to accept who you are. Everyone has darkness and light. Visit the temple and say, "I accept who I am now, including my darkness."

The Temple of Beauty: You can go to the Temple of Beauty to learn to appreciate your life and to see the beauty in it. Rather than seeing everyday life as dull, you appreciate that your life is charming from the time you wake up in the morning. Visit the temple and say, "I am ready for life. It is not dull anymore."

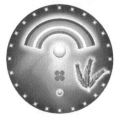

The Temple of Wisdom: There are three types of wisdom: lower wisdom from the personality, higher wisdom from the soul, and super higher wisdom from your mighty I Am presence. You must start integrating this higher wisdom now.

Going to this temple can be very supportive,

especially for ascension, because the more wisdom you gain, the more karmic energy you will release without having to go through physical experiences of living that karma. Karma is about energy balance and gaining wisdom. The more wisdom you have, the more karma is released.

The Temple of Knowingness: This temple is where you experience your existence not as a concept but as a reality. When you go to this temple, ask that this awareness be awakened so that you can integrate it and "know" as an experience.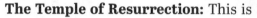

The Temple of Resurrection: This is the temple where you can resurrect any aspect of your life. You can resurrect the wisdom of your soul, the support of your guides, and the Creator's energy. You must resurrect and re-create daily, monthly, or at least every three months. It is called resetting your energies.

You must reset your energies for higher frequencies. For example, you do not watch much television, but you watch Gaia TV, is that true?

Correct.

Because you don't feel resonance with other television?

Oh, no, it's awful.

Exactly. In a way, you have reset that energy. Look at the books you read. They are not like those you read ten years ago. You do not read those books because they do not have the same frequency you now have. You are a higher being. You do not interact with the same people because you have a higher vibration. You interact with like-minded people. That is why it is very important to reset your energy at least every three months. During meditation, you can say, "I reset (or recalibrate) my energy with the new consciousness of who I am today." You are not who you were last fall. You have already grown from summer to fall. This is an important process.

The Temple of Release: This is where you can release petty things in life, like jealousy, gossip, and everyday worries.

The Temple of Expansion: This is where you can ask to expand in any area of your life — an energy, an experience, or a thought, anything you want to expand. Go to this temple during meditation or set the intention to visit there before you go to sleep, and ask for what you want to be expanded. For example, you could ask that your divine creativity, divine abundance, or divine connection with like-minded people be expanded.

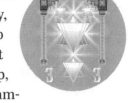

The Temple of Healing: This temple is for all types of healing. You can visit this temple to heal past and present belief systems that affect your mental, emotional, and spiritual bodies. When you go to this temple, you cleanse yourself at every level so that your aura becomes purified. Your aura must have absolute purity for ascension. When you work at this temple, your aura becomes very clear and pure.

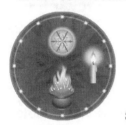

Temple of the Violet Flame: The violet flame is used for transmuting energies of the Earth plane, as well as other planes, of past lives and cellular imprints. You can set the intention to visit this temple while you sleep. Say, "I ask my guides to safely take me to the Temple of the Violet Flame so that I can purify myself."

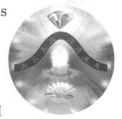

The Temple of Jade: Taoists and Buddhists know about this temple. They go there regularly to partake of the ancient wisdom of the East, which comes directly from the Central Sun. Say, "I go to the Temple of Jade to purify and to integrate higher wisdom into my being."

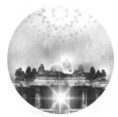

Confucianism, Taoism, and other mystical religions and teachings come from other planetary realities. The energy of the Central Sun carries the frequency and thought patterns of all the masters from Earth as well as other dimensions, galaxies, and planetary systems. We strongly recommend going to the Temple of Jade.

The Ashram of Archangel Michael: The Ashram of Archangel Michael sits atop a crystal mountain. This place is visited by many ascended masters and other planetary beings. Working with the dense energy of the Earth plane also affects the masters, so they go there to rejuvenate.

The Crystal Temple on Arcturus: Visit this temple before you go to sleep. Ask to lie on the crystal bed. Imagine you are filled with crystalline light and purified. Simply asking that this be done during sleep is all that is needed. You can ask to be purified daily. You will slowly see your life becoming more sacred and more loving. You will be in harmony within, and your aura will become stronger.

The Temple of Integration: When you visit this temple (and any of the other temples) during meditation or in your sleep, hold the intention to be able to integrate all the energies available for your spiritual evolution.

The Temple of Merging: The temple of merging allows you to integrate three aspects of you — the soul, the monad, and the I Am presence. For our purposes, "merging" means rejoining.

The Temple of Re-creation: While you visit the Temple of Re-creation, you can ask to re-create any part of your life you would like to manifest in your present reality. When you make a statement in this temple, part of your akash (which contains the limitations of your present life) is released, and the memories that contain benevolence will become part of your reality. For instance, you all carry energetic imprints of trauma in your akash, but it also contains positive, benevolent imprints from the forefront of your consciousness. Your lives are run by the memories contained in your cellular structure.

The Temple of Mastery: When you visit the Temple of Mastery, you can request mastery of any limitations you are facing, such as thought patterns and belief systems.

Comets and Solar Flares

We will take some questions now, dear brother.

Thank you. This question is about some of the spiritual superstars in the United States — David Wilcock,[1] Corey Goode, and a man who calls himself Cobra, from the Pleiades. There are others as well. These people speak of ascension as an event that is triggered by a solar flare that will shift the energy of the solar system and lift humans to a higher state of consciousness. They call this solar flare "the event." As I understand it, the conception of ascension is a more passive situation, not based on individual effort as much as being present when the event happens. Would you comment on this please?

Yes, it is true. Intense solar energy is bombarding the planet at this time. This is why you see so much turmoil, because of the intensity. It is a purification energy, for there is a potential for a comet to hit Earth in another two-and-a-half to three years.

Angels and other beings are doing an enormous amount of work to deflect this comet because if it hits the planet, there would be a great cataclysm. There would be a great flux, and many cities would be affected. But angels are working to deflect this comet from hitting Africa, which would cause damages all over America.

Because the intensity of the solar flares is increasing, people are becoming more purified and refined. The more people awaken, the more this comet can be deflected. Having said that, we believe that all people must take responsibility for themselves by creating their luminous bodies. The planet will support this through the intense flares. But will humanity be lifted up solely by the flares? From our viewpoint, no. However, human beings will be very much supported if they put in the effort. The solar flares will increase.

There is great change happening on Earth. There has been a great shift in the polar icecaps. A huge portion of ice has broken and is now floating in the ocean. If it melts in the ocean, the water will rise, and many cities could be flooded.

Yes, I have heard of this. This is part of the Antarctic icecap that is about to let go.

There is great work being done by angels to deflect the disaster this could create, and solar flares are making people become more conscious of their choices. They are becoming aware they need to take responsibility by pumping the energy of naturalness into them. From our viewpoint, humanity will not be lifted en masse. They will

---

1.   Learn more about David Wilcock at https://www.gaia.com/person/david-wilcock.

have to work this out for themselves. But it will become easier to do as more people awaken, and this energy will spread.

The first people who do this, presumably the readers of this book, will be the way-showers to make it easier for other people to follow. Is that true?

It will not only be the people who read this book. Some people already had ascension energy after 2012. More than 3 million people already have ascension energy integrated. Right now there are many people experiencing ascension, and by 2030, there will be at least 33 million more, and they will all be supporting this shift. By simply being present and aware, you are supporting the energy shift.

For example, imagine you are going to a supermarket. Your light is also going there. Do you think you're just buying some bread? No, you're bringing light to the supermarket. But we bless brother Wilcock, for he is an ancient soul. He is trying to do what is best (from his point of view) to lift humanity, so we honor him for that.

I have nothing but respect. Much of his work is amazing. I think what I'm questioning is the concept that humans will go up in a huge "poof!" with the solar event that is going to lift all humanity. There's no hard work in that.

He's going to become more famous and, of course, more controversial, but many will follow him, and they will see some interesting revelations coming up, for there will be a time coming when you will discover some new pyramids on the planet.

I read the other day about one in the Bermuda Triangle. They found something in Antarctica too, this sort of thing.

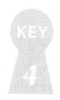

Integrate Galactic Consciousness

The Family of God, Master Chao, and Master Mahareya

The Family of God: Hello, brother Robert. We are the Family of God. It is always a joyous moment when our hearts are connected with your heart and the hearts of humanity. We bring love, grace, and peace to your heart. Be still, and enjoy these feelings for a moment before we begin.

Rae asked that we bring understanding about the keys to your evolution so that you can join with the light that you are. Ascension key 4 is about galactic remembrances, the integration of galactic consciousness. You did not originate from Earth but from another reality. This has been mentioned many times and in many writings. If you do not know where you came from, you cannot go where you want to go. Understanding your past is very important so that you can understand where you came from as you journey on the Earth plane.

There are many levels of galactic consciousness you must access, experience, understand, and integrate. The first level of galactic consciousness is the Adam consciousness. Adam and Eve were the perfect humans designed to carry out the will of the Creator by the Creator.

The Adam code exists in every human being, and it is situated in the pineal gland, in the middle of the medulla oblongata.

The Adam code has also been called the signature code, or the signature cell, but we do not believe this terminology is correct. We call the Adam code the God code, for Adam was designed in the image and perfection of the Creator.

You can connect with the Adam code within you by awakening your pineal gland. This is why it is so important to focus on the pineal gland: Breathe into it, communicate with it, activate it, and integrate its energy throughout your being.

A human being is not just an Earth being. In reality, humans are universal beings. Later in the evolution of humanity, you will not be called Earth citizens but rather galactic citizens.

You must integrate different levels of galactic energy, and this starts with integrating the energy of planet Earth. The master who supports and holds the frequency for Earth is Master Buddha, for he is the planetary guardian. Master Melchior is the master of galactic consciousness. The masters who can help you integrate solar consciousness are Masters Helio and Vesta. Lord Melchizedek is the master of universal consciousness, applicable to the universe you are in now. The master of multiuniversal wisdom, energy, and consciousness is Archangel Metatron.

The next level of galactic consciousness is murion consciousness, and the master to connect with this is Master Chao. To connect with this consciousness, simply call it forward. Then you must connect with the Great Central Sun consciousness. The Great Central Sun represents the wisdom, love, and heart process energy of all the masters for all these universes combined in an energetic form. Simply said, the Central Sun contains energy of all the masters throughout all levels we have mentioned thus far. Then you must integrate the energy of Mahatma. The Mahatma energy is next to us, the Family of God. Mahatma energy supports humanity's evolution.

Integrate the Different Dimensions of Consciousness

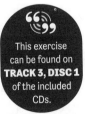

This exercise can be found on **TRACK 3, DISC 1** of the included CDs.

1. The first dimension of consciousness to integrate is the Earth heart, the physical heart. Visualize the shape of a heart made of flowers in front of the area

of your physical heart (where the etheric, or interdimensional, heart resides). It is a beautiful, pale-brown earth color.

2. Visualize that 1 foot behind this heart is the galactic heart. It is a shiny copper.
3. Visualize that 1 foot behind the galactic heart is the solar heart. It is pale white, and it is also made of flowers.
4. Behind that, you see the universal heart. It is a beautiful silver and is also made of flowers.
5. Visualize that 1 foot behind that is the multiuniversal heart in shining platinum.
6. The murion heart is behind that, and it is a beautiful metallic-blue made of flowers.
7. Behind that is the Central Sun heart. It is a beautiful gold.
8. Behind the Central Sun heart is the energy of the Mahatma heart. It is a beautiful turquoise.
9. Visualize that you are passing a needle and thread through all these hearts, joining them. Once they are strung together, tie the ends of the thread to your heart. On the left side of your heart will be the planetary heart. On the right side of your heart will be the Mahatma heart.
10. Breathe into the planetary heart. See your breath going through all these hearts and coming back to you with the energy of the Mahatma heart filling you. You might feel expansion in your heart. Breathe, breathe, and continuously breathe.
11. Visualize two hearts expanding, one on either side of you. You are in the middle. Just keep breathing. Keep breathing.
12. You can make this sound: "Lannot kiyaeum, lannot kiyaeum, lannot kiyaeum." This means, "I speak the voice of God through all my realities."

When you do this exercise once a day for a minimum of 30 days, you will be able to integrate this consciousness. It is in your being, and you will carry this consciousness always. You will feel these hearts beat inside you. This means you have embraced your entire past from the galactic consciousness. Your consciousness exists in all these realities. These realities have masters. You will be able to connect and integrate the energy of these masters within you.

What will happen when you follow this practice for 30 days? Your body will feel warm. You might feel a cauldron of fire on the top of your head, and this fire warms you. It emits a beautiful, soft-white light. Your personal wisdom pours into you. You will awaken all your bodies through all times and realities because galactic consciousness exists throughout all times and realities.

Restore Your Essence

Human beings have been genetically manipulated to keep them in darkness. You have chakras on the outside of your wrists called ancestral chakras. They are also called ancestral memory chakras because they contain the memory of who you are. This has been wiped from your memory bank. With this practice, you will be healed, and these hooks will be released. You will remember more of yourself. When you begin this practice, you will feel a bit uncomfortable. You will feel as if you are carrying flowers on both sides of your body with a feeling of lightness but some uneasiness too.

How will you know you have become fully integrated? You will start smelling the flowers. When you smell the flowers, you will know you have joined with the many other galactic parts of your consciousness. Now, we invite the great Master Chao along with Master Mahareya to speak with you.

Connect with Lightbeing Consciousness

Master Chao and Master Mahareya: Hello, my brother and the family of humanity. It is very important to understand your origin. Through all these dimensions, human beings have had lives not as human beings but as lightbeings and sometimes just as particles of light. Just one drop of light contains your whole essence.

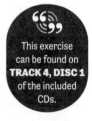

This exercise can be found on **TRACK 4, DISC 1** of the included CDs.

1. Please close your eyes. You have visualized putting the thread through each heart, and you have imagined all these hearts. Visualize them again now.

2. Now add a beautiful silver spark of light, a small dot, or a silver sparkle going from your physical heart through the first, the second, the third, the fourth, the fifth, the sixth, the seventh, and the eighth hearts. It is like a beam of light going around and coming

back into your physical heart. Just breathe in this light. This light will increase in intensity and also in volume. This point of light will become bigger and bigger. You are stringing all the hearts together through your light.

3. Now inwardly say, "Lannot kiyaeum, lannot kiyaeum, lannot kiyaeum." See this sound go into the middle of each heart and come back to your heart. Say: "Lannot kiyaeum, lannot kiyaeum, lannot kiyaeum."

4. You might see sparks go through the hearts, burning like a beautiful garland of fire. "Lannot kiyaeum, lannot kiyaeum."

5. This fire will go to the top of your head and shine light. "Lannot kiyaeum, lannot kiyaeum, lannot kiyaeum." You are integrating your galactic consciousness, and many karmic energies brought forth from these realities will be healed during this meditation technique. They will lose their potential to manifest because the higher energy will dilute these karmic energies, and they will be dissolved and released.

6. Now form a mudra [figure 4.1]: Open your hands with your fingers touching, including your thumbs. Place your left hand on your solar plexus. Place your right hand on your heart. Just breathe it in.

7. Chant: "Lannot kiyaeum, lannot kiyaeum, lannot kiyaeum."

This mudra and chant will help you find your galactic consciousness and fully integrate it within you. We suggest doing this once a day for 30 days for maximum results.

I am Master Chao along with Master Mahareya.

Family of God: "Lannot kiyaeum" means "I integrate my galactic consciousness from all realities, and I speak from that voice from now onward." When you chant this, you might feel energy in your forehead, not only in your third eye, but also above it.

Yes, I do. From my conception as a physical human being, I see galactic consciousness as relating to the galaxy that I live in, which is the Milky Way. Does this consciousness extend beyond that? Am I limiting galactic consciousness through my conception of seeing it as this galaxy?

There are many galaxies.

I know.

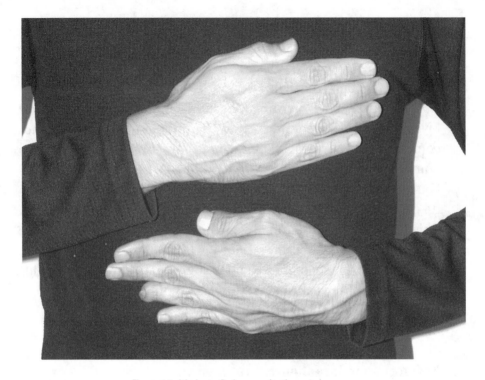

Figure 4.1. Mudra to find your galactic consciousness

But you are not able to see them, so don't limit this. Simply say, "I gather all of my galactic consciousness."

Right, so this pertains not only to this galaxy. It is for all galaxies?

Yes, because you are coming to the place of the universe, not just one galaxy. The universe contains many galaxies.

Yes, and it contains many dimensions. So does this include all dimensions?

Yes, exactly.

My second question is about the Mahatma level. Is Mahatma the master of that level?

Yes, Mahatma is a master of that level. Mahatma is the one who brings the energy from the Family of God and distributes it throughout all realities and to the Earth plane. For example, why should you integrate energies of Master Buddha? Because Master Buddha is a planetary guardian on the Earth's physical plane, and you have lives on Earth's physical plane. You should integrate the energy of Lord Melchizedek because he is the master of this universe. There are many universes, but he is the master of the universe of which Earth is a part. You see?

Yes, okay.

In the same way, Mahatma is the consciousness who dilutes the energy of the Creator and brings it into this reality and this universe.

Okay.

You and the readers of this book are now undertaking a PhD. There will be many mentors who will guide you through certain steps. Perhaps a Buddhist mentor will take you to one level for the first six months and the next mentor will take you to the next level and so forth. They are guides who can support you at each level to go to the next level.

Understood.

All are important.

Okay, I think I'm getting the picture now. We are being restored to our pure essence.

Of course, ascension is only that. You are coming back to yourself once again.

Activate the Ascension Codes

The Family of God

Family of God: Hello, we are the Family of God. Ascension key 5 is about activating ascension codes located in your higher chakras. You are aware of the seven chakras, and you are aware of the eighth chakra, the soul star chakra, which is about 8 to 10 inches above your head. It is a beautiful silver color. You are also aware of the ninth chakra, the earth-star chakra, which is 8 to 10 inches beneath your feet.

There are codes of ascensions in your tenth, twelfth, twenty-first, thirty-third, and forty-forth chakras, and this key is about activating those codes. Each of these chakras has a color and a numeric code. Each is overseen by a master who can help you activate its codes.

The tenth chakra is 12 to 15 inches above your head. It is called the harhom chakra, and it contains Earth codes. It is white. When these codes are activated, your life on Earth becomes easy. You are able to see the patterns of your life, how you have set up your contract for greatest growth, and how you will be able to create much more.

Most people are only vaguely aware of their contracts in life. They do not have a very clear picture at all. When your tenth chakra is fully activated, the understanding and remembrance of your life contract makes every aspect of your life much easier. Your blueprint becomes clearer, and it is easier for you to take action. You can call on Master Chao to help you integrate these codes. The numeric code for the tenth chakra is 97.

The twelfth chakra is called the yamne chakra. It is approximately one arm's length above your head. Its color is blue, and you can call on Master Arhimi to help you with this chakra. The numeric code is 121.

The twenty-first chakra extends 8 inches behind your shoulder blade. It is called the high heart chakra or the vijram chakra. Its color is turquoise. You can call on Master Malaya for help with this chakra. The numeric code is 212.

The thirty-third chakra is called the Adam Kadmon chakra. It is a beautiful golden star. It is located about 10 feet above your head. Archangel Metatron can help you with this chakra. The numeric code is 316.

The forty-fourth chakra is called the myro chakra. This chakra exists in two places, about 30 feet in front of you and 30 feet behind you. Its color is translucent white. Two masters can help you with this chakra: Master Mahareya and Master Poohali. The numeric code for this chakra is 514.

Chakras with Ascension Activation Codes

Higher Chakras	Tenth	Twelfth	Twenty-First	Thirty-Third	Forty-Fourth
Name	Harhom	Yamne	Vijram	Adam Kadmon	Myro
Location	12–15 in. above head	arm's length above head	8 in. behind shoulder blade	10 ft. above head	30 ft. front & back
Color	white	blue	turquoise	golden star	translucent white
Master	Chao	Arhimi	Malaya	Archangel Metatron	Mahareya & Poohali
Code	97	121	212	316	514

Exercises to Activate Your Ascension Codes

Focus on the area of the tenth chakra, 12 to 15 inches above your head. Close your eyes, and say, "97, 97, 97, 97, 97, 97, 97."

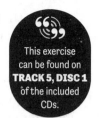

This exercise can be found on **TRACK 5, DISC 1** of the included CDs.

Ninety-seven, 97, 97, 97, 97. I can feel it starting to activate. I'm feeling a sensation up there.

You will see some colors fall down your twelfth chakra and go through your entire body and into the ground. Say, "97," and then you will go deeper and deeper into yourself. Say, "97, 97, 97, 97." Do this for 5 minutes.

It feels as if I'm being washed with ... it feels like a whitish light.

Beautiful. Now we will go to the next one. Take your awareness to the twelfth chakra, which is approximately one arm's length above you, and say, "121 (one twenty-one), 121, 121, 121, 121, 121." You might feel energy falling, and you might feel a shiver or goose bumps. It will come over you like a waterfall from this twelfth chakra. Say, "121, 121, 121, 121, 121, 121, 121, 121, 121, 121, 121, 121." Continue to say this for 5 minutes.

I feel it. It's blue, and I feel a strange tingling going on.

Yes. You can feel energy coming down over you.

Yes, I do.

Now, go to the back of the body to the area where the heart is, and make the statement: "212 (two twelve) 212, 212, 212, 212, 212." You might feel some odd sensations in your stomach or at the front of your body. Say, "212, 212, 212, 212." Say this for 5 minutes.

To me, it feels as if I'm moving into something else.

Exactly. You are opening, and you're joining your quantum being.

Yes, wow.

Now, imagine, to the best of your ability, the Adam Kadmon (thirty-third) chakra, which is located about 10 feet above your head. Say, "316 (three sixteen) 316, 316, 316, 316." Let's do this for 5 minutes: "316. 316, 316, 316." You might feel some pressure on your eyebrows or your third eye: "316, 316." You might feel some pounding energy, or you might see fire coming in: "316, 316, 316, 316, 316, 316, 316, 316, 316."

I can feel it coming into me, and it's making my body go into small spasms, little convulsions, nothing serious. It's like my body is accepting this energy with a small shudder.

Now, the next one is the forty-fourth chakra, which is 30 feet in front and behind you. This time let's call Master Mahareya. Say, "Master Mahareya, I am ready to accept this light into me." When you make the statement, say, "514 (five fourteen), 514, 514." You will see this 514 extend and go inside you: "514, 514, 514, 514, 514, 514, 514, 514, 514, 514." Sometimes you might even feel a string is going through you: "514." Say this for 5 minutes.

I think I feel a bit of ... it's making me shudder a little bit, but it's very beautiful. It's like, from the way I feel this, it's some place else. I know there's a part of me that's a little afraid of it, but it's very beautiful. It's beautiful.

This contains special codes, and you can feel the energy. So we suggest that the people working on ascension tone these numbers. They can also call on the masters, visualize the color, and then tone these numbers. The numbers have energy frequencies in them along with a geometric pattern. All will be downloaded into you, and your ascension codes will be activated.

It's very beautiful. In doing these exercises, should someone work on one chakra, one code, at a time? Or would it be appropriate to do all five of them in one sitting?

Do one at a time, and spend about 5 minutes on each.

So they need to commit themselves to about 25 minutes to do these exercises.

We only ask people for three years of their entire lifetimes to do this work to achieve ascension. This is for those on a fast track. They should do these exercises for 30 to 45 days. Those who are really dedicated will take the time to do it.

Connect with the Earth Spirit

The Family of God

Family of God: We are the family of God. Our blessings and love to you. Today we bring some understanding for ascension key 6 regarding Earth and its connection to the human body. The elements that make up Earth are the same elements in your body. This is common knowledge, but what is not understood is that your body is much more than these elements, and Earth is much more than these elements.

The Earth spirit is a living, breathing being, just like you, but her physical structure is different from yours. She breathes, and if you are sensitive, you will be able to hear the sound of her heartbeat. Many clairvoyant people are able to tune in to Earth and feel her love.

Your body and your soul contain the very essence of the Earth spirit. What does this mean? Some of the components used to make your soul energy include the elements of the Earth spirit along with other planetary bodies. This means that your soul is made up of many materials, including the consciousness of some masters. You could call this the skin of your soul. Other components in your soul include the planets and galaxies that are directly interrelated to Earth.

The Earth spirit holds many codes pertaining to human beings, animals, plants, and heavenly bodies. There are many codes. The Earth spirit is continuously communing with other realities, dimensions, galaxies, and planets. When you awaken the Earth code within you, you will be able to tap into the other realities that the Earth spirit communicates and communes with.

The Earth spirit is known by many names in many cultures. We would like to give you one of her spiritual names. This spiritual name is Aram Ii Am. The last part of her name is pronounced "m."

The Earth spirit holds the code of ascension in this reality. Human beings have made soul contracts to work in this reality, because here you will be able to fully awaken your energy and attain liberation. The Earth spirit always presents this reality to your face. You could say that you want to run away from this world, that you don't feel connected to it, and that you don't feel you belong here. The Earth spirit always presents the Earth reality to you, gently reminding you that this is the place you have come and this is the place you must be. It is through this place that you will work toward liberation or ascension. No matter how you try to avoid it, the Earth spirit pushes this reality in front of you. You cannot push it aside. It is always in front of you. Wouldn't you agree, brother?

Yes. It is set up so that we can liberate ourselves. It's a school for that purpose.

Yes. You will be liberated through this Earth reality. You are here at this moment. Your liberation will not happen through any other reality except the Earth reality.

Right. If we don't make it this time, we get the opportunity to come back. Is that correct?

You will. You will have the opportunity to come back and do it again but only in this reality. It is important to remember that this is your present reality, and you cannot escape it. It will be presented to you. It will chase you all over. So it is best to accept that this is the reality through which you are going to work for liberation. It also holds the codes for your ascension.

Activate the Earth Spirit Codes

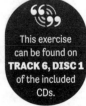

This exercise can be found on **TRACK 6, DISC 1** of the included CDs.

1. Visualize two twirling golden spheres, each 1 foot in diameter, extending from your navel, one in front of the other.

2. Breathe from your navel, and send energy to these

spheres. Send energy from your navel to these spheres in the pattern of an infinity symbol.

3. Breathe into them, and see the infinity symbol multiply. There are many infinity symbols that extend from your navel to these spheres and come back to you. The infinity symbol surrounds the spheres. Just breathe it in.

4. The Earth spirit master is named Master Rahimi. Now, let us call this master by saying three times, "Rahimi. Rahimi. Rahimi."

5. Visualize this master standing between the two spheres. He has a beard and is wearing white clothes and a golden cap.

6. This master will touch the infinity symbol between the two spheres and tone the sound "sarhom, sarhom, sarhom."

7. When he makes this sound, golden light comes from his fingers into the infinity symbol and into the two spheres: "sarhom, sarhom, sarhom."

8. You might feel warmth in your stomach area. You might also feel energy moving. Just stay in this space: "sarhom, sarhom."

9. Tone this three times: "sarhom, sarhom, sarhom. Sarhom, sarhom, sarhom. Sarhom, sarhom, sarhom."

10. You will now receive geometric patterns coming from the infinity symbol and the spheres. Do not open your eyes. These sacred geometric patterns come from the master's hands: tetrahedron, hexahedron, octahedron, dodecahedron, icosahedron, triangle, and circle. These sacred geometric patterns flow from the master's hands into the infinity symbol, into the sphere, and into you.

11. See yourself inside these sacred geometric patterns — the triangle, circle, tetrahedron, hexahedron, octahedron, dodecahedron, icosahedron. Breathe it in. Breathe it in. You are inside these geometric patterns. The codes for ascension are in these sacred geometric patterns. See these codes coming into you with the geometric patterns. Just breathe this.

12. Slowly these geometric patterns will expand around you, from beneath your feet and over your head, and now you are inside the geometric patterns. The geometric patterns are the design of the universe, and once you finish the basic level of the chakras, you operate through sacred geometry and codes. Just breathe it in.

13. You will see some glistening colors appear on the sacred geometric

patterns. Some will be gold. Some will be metallic colors. Some will be orange. Any color is okay.

14. The geometric patterns are spinning now, some clockwise and some counterclockwise — spinning, spinning, spinning, and downloading energies into not only your physical body but also your auric body, which contains many codes of ascension.

15. Now you will see some numbers falling from these geometric patterns. There are numbers all around you. The number could be 1, 6, or 9. Just breathe it in.

16. Now make this statement: "I hold the frequency of my ascension within me now." Breathe deeply.

17. Open your palms, and some of the sacred geometric patterns might appear on your hands, dancing and creating energy and bringing pure light.

18. Now chant, "Sarhom," slowly. These patterns in your hands will spin very fast. "Sarhom, sarhom, sarhom. Sarhom, sarhom, sarhom. Sarhom, sarhom, sarhom. Sarhom, sarhom, sarhom."

19. See these geometric patterns completely embedded within you. You are a walking geometric form now. Breathe in and out three times. See it become embedded within you. You will carry these codes in you from now on, and you become aware of your codes.

These codes are activated by two simple qualities you can cultivate — love and laughter. When you truly laugh, these codes vibrate. These codes can also be activated using certain sound frequencies (especially some ancient choral music), certain smells, the energy of the Moon, and the early sunrise. Any kind of honoring choral music is appropriate, such as something sung by the Mormon Tabernacle Choir. Just breathe it in.

From now on, you carry a big responsibility. You carry the ascension codes. Be aware of it. Just become aware of these codes, moment to moment. You will start feeling this energy. Sometimes you might feel a tingling sensation when they come into you.

Tone: "Sarhom, sarhom, yahe. Me ue shumm. Ta na ua tusu. Umm myo yii. Umm myo yii. Umm myo yin. Umm myo yii. Umm myo yii. Umm, myo yin." This is a galactic language. When you tone the last three sounds, you will feel some energy in your brain, in the middle of your head. "Umm myo yin, umm myo yin, umm myo yin" is a seed mantra. If you tone this, it will open you to a higher reality. It will take you deeper and deeper, and you will merge into eternal consciousness.

Sound: "umm myo yii, umm myo yii, umm myo yin." These tones are sung and sounded, not spoken. Then after singing, stay in meditation for a minimum of 10 minutes with this energy and sound. It will go into your body.

Tomorrow when you wake up and you're sitting with your cat, scratch his head and make the sound "umm myo yin." It acts just as a seed, and this seed will go deeper and deeper. Within 5 minutes, you will feel you are in a deep state of relaxation, and sometimes you will see that in your inner space. Find your own way of toning. There's no one correct way: "umm myo yin."

Do this once a day for 10 minutes for at least 90 days.

$\mathscr{P}$urify $\mathscr{L}$ayers of $\mathscr{T}$hought

The Family of God

Family of God: Ascension key 7 is about understanding what purification truly means. There is a master from Arcturus associated with purification: Na Ha Mo Ch. Arcturus is the stargate for your ascension and a portal for ascension. It is an important midway point between the Great Central Sun and planet Earth. There are wise beings on Arcturus who support humanity.

Purification involves many things. We are not talking about purifying the body. Most of you take care of that on some level. We are talking about purification of the mind, the soul, the mental body, the emotional body, and the spiritual body, as well as your relationship to Earth and your connection with the elements. All these need to be purified. When this is done, purification occurs on many levels, including the karmic and ancestral levels.

True purification comes first in the mind. Your thought process supports the manifestation of your reality. Thoughts are divided into many layers, up to eight. For example, what was the thought you heard first when you entered the Earth plane as you were born? Was it a thought you picked up from a doctor? Thoughts are energy forms, and you might have absorbed the sound frequency of the energy coming as a word as well as anxiety, fear, or something else. This is very important. We must heal first thoughts, what you first heard as a baby.

In the Islamic culture, as soon as newborns are washed, they are given to the fathers to hold. The father whispers the name of Allah in the child's ear.

The second level of thought that a child picks up is from the interaction of its parents, especially during the first three to six months. Thoughts are also picked up from the grandparents and other relatives. The third level of thought is when a caregiver reads storybooks, sings songs, or rocks the baby. The baby picks up thoughts from this about the stories and the words in the books. These imprint on the baby's mind.

The fourth level of thought is formed when the child goes out into the world for the first time and is exposed to other children. This could start in kindergarten or daycare. It usually starts when the child is four to five years old. These imprints are much stronger. The child meets other children. There is anxiety and fear in being separated from the parents. The child thinks, "I have to trust the unknown and the teacher here." The child is very aware but not able to communicate. There are other students, and many might be from past lives. So there is great fear. Many children will not let go of their parents' hands, and they cry because of anxiety and fear. All this plays a very big role throughout their lives.

The fifth level of thought happens when a person starts to feel a strong physical and emotional attraction to someone else. When people start liking each other, these thoughts are very powerful. A boy could say, "You are very beautiful. You are very special to me." The word "special" goes very deep into a girl, and she could say, "I love you." This is very powerful. It's the first time she has heard it from a boy she likes, and he hears it too. A very strong emotion is activated at that time.

The sixth level of thought is formed when a person enters the workplace. There are many thoughts from other beings in the work environment. This has a big effect on the psyche and how a person perceives and interacts with people not only in the work environment but also during later stages of life.

The seventh level of thought with a very big impact is when people say "I do" to get married. Then the eighth level is when they have children. All these thoughts affect one's being.

There are many other thoughts — cultural thoughts, thoughts about the family's needs, thoughts about one's country, and thoughts about others' opinions. But the thoughts we have mentioned have a profound influence on the body. The person who wants to ascend must purify these thoughts.

Healing Begins at Your Energetic Conception

The starting point of a human life is the moment the parents first look at each other. They are not in love. They just look at each other and feel a similarity: "I want to get to know this person." And that is the moment the baby's energy is conceived. They might have sexual union later — get married and have children — but the point of origin of a baby is in that moment of first meeting. So healing must begin at that point.

When sexual union happens, the baby picks up all the mother's fears at that time. You must heal that moment as well. The father's sperm is very intelligent. Millions of sperm race toward the waiting egg, and the mother is waiting. Out of millions of sperm, only one sperm makes life. This sperm has intelligence. It has consciousness. It needs to go to the mother's waiting egg. So healing that sperm must take place at that moment. This is not very difficult.

Once you understand the concept, you will see that it is rather simple. Healing must take place first in thought. These thoughts carry the imprints of the belief systems of the people around the parents. Next, you need to heal the belief systems. Thoughts and belief systems are very important. Master Na Ha Mo Ch from Arcturus can help you heal them. When these two aspects are healed, many other aspects of energy that are layered on top of them will lose their grip.

Purification Exercise

1. Call on the great master Na Ha Mo Ch: "I call on the master Na Ha Mo Ch from the benevolent planet Arcturus. I ask to be taken to the temple of Myo." Myo is the mother of Arcturus. The master will take you to this temple.

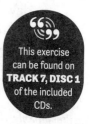

This exercise can be found on **TRACK 7, DISC 1** of the included CDs.

2. Ask the master to pour pure water on the top of your head. Visualize the liquid being poured over your head.

3. Now make this statement: "I immerse myself in this holy and sacred water, and I release all my thoughts and belief systems that no longer serve me in integrating the light of ascension within me."

4. Visualize bubbles of light in many shades of gray falling from your body and your auric field. See them float away like dull gray clouds. This exercise is best done for 20 minutes.

5. Once this is complete, ask the goddess Myo to take you to the purification chamber. There is a beautiful, sacred platinum fire. Sit in front of this fire for 20 minutes, and chant this song three times: "Ma hi yo ma ua. Sa hi va. Me vya. San ho ti. Ne me ai. Sans, sans, sans." Chant it three more times: "Ma hi yo ma ua. Sa hi va. Me vya. San ho ti. Ne me ai. Sans, sans, sans." Don't open your eyes. Make these sounds in your own way: "San ho ti. San ho ti. San ho ti. San ho ti."

   These sounds cleanse your organs, tissues, bloodstream, bones, kidneys, and heart. Your physical body holds many karmic imprints. When a thought imprints, the experience imprints. All is held in the physical body — the skin, hair, nails, and auric field. When you make these sounds, you are asking to cleanse all that your physical body contains. This will also purify ancestral belief systems preventing you from moving forward.

6. The great Arcturian master of music Vasha Kai walks in. He gives you a seed sound. He whispers in your ear, and you make this sound silently: "room ba, room ba." Just chant this quietly. This seed sound will take you deeper and deeper into yourself, and you will be immersed in the eternal consciousness for about 10 minutes. "Room ba, room ba, room ba room, room, room."

7. This purification exercise must be done daily for a minimum of 90 days and then once a week. You can even call this the mother of purification because this process encompasses all lifetimes as well as your bodily organs, past karmic energies, ancestral energies, star energies from other planets, star karma, country karma, lineage karma, and cultural karma. Everything is lifted.

Presumably, these will shift around during the 90-day period?

Yes, you will see differently. You will feel liberated: "I am a little bit more free in my mind and in my heart."

These keys should be done in sequence, if I am correct. So the first thing to do is the twenty-one days of clearing the aura, of uniting the aura?

It is good to do these in sequence, but an experienced student might move through these differently. A beginner will want to work in sequence, but people who have been on the path for a while can just pick up where they feel appropriate and work from there.

Okay, so it's okay to jump around for people who are more advanced?

Exactly. The only thing we tell advanced people is to at least learn about auric cleansing. It is very important.

Right. Well, I'm definitely starting with that.

Remember Your Origin

How do you define ascension? What is it in your words?

This is a very good question. We say ascension is simply remembrances of your origin and being able to bring these remembrances into the present, along with the energy of the remembrances from all realities, times, and spaces. So you might ask, "What is the purpose of life?" It is to remember who you are and to express these remembrances in every moment. It also means, "I have come here to join with the god/goddess that I am, and I am able to express this god/goddess moment to moment in every experience I create and re-create." This is a very simple explanation. Does it make some sense to you?

It does. It is beautiful in its simplicity. I like it so much.

You can also say that remembrance means you remember who you are. So who are you? You are a light unto yourself. Remembrance also means your cells remember everything. What do they remember? They remember light, and every cell vibrates with the remembrance that you are the light. We are the light.

"Ascension" is just a word. It means "remembrances of the light," and you experience this light every moment through every cell of your body. So you do not want to emphasize the word "ascension." Many people associate light with ascension. So we allow that to happen, and that's all. You will see when you grow that you will not use the word "ascension." You will use the word "light": "I am the light, and I express this light." Jesus never mentioned ascension. He only mentioned light and love.

But it also amounts to returning to Source in consciousness, I would say.

Yes. Yes. Of course. It's returning to the Source, returning to oneness, and returning to the remembrance of who you are.

Which is really the moment of creation of individual souls.

Exactly. Coming home to yourself. Look at the word "remembrance." If you divide the word "remember," what does it mean? Re-member. You are returning to be a member of the family of God once again. You see the difference?

Yes, I do.

Re-membering yourself. And who are you? The Family of God.

Hmm. Well, it's beautiful. Thank you. That's lovely. There are other things too, like having access to past and future incarnations and moving away from linear time. But those are side effects. You've nailed it very well.

There is a lot of information available on all subjects, and we want to bring something completely new to people. We also tell people, all that you are doing is thirty-three keys, and if you feel inspired, read other books, because there is more wisdom that can support you. This book itself is enough, but be on the lookout for other tools that might benefit you.

Purification is quite difficult. Purification of the mind is not difficult compared to purification of belief systems. This is very difficult. Beliefs are based on ideological concepts, and they are very difficult to break. Take the Islamic terrorists who have killed people. They are good people, but they are fighting for an ideology, only an ideology. They don't hate the people they kill, but they believe in an ideal. You see the difference, brother?

I do. I understand.

An ideology is very difficult to break.

All the "isms."

Exactly. One of the ideologies many men carry is that women are supposed to be child bearers, cook the food, and take care of the children. They consider women as second-class citizens in the world, that their role is in the house with the children. Many cultures still carry this.

Connect All Realities

The Family of God

Family of God: We are the Family of God. Our love surrounds you and your house. We send you protection for your house and your small creatures. Today, we wish to talk about ascension key 8. This key represents the connection of all realities, or you could simply say all our perspectives.

Link to Your Quantum Body

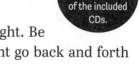

This exercise can be found on **TRACK 8, DISC 1** of the included CDs.

1. See yourself in a cube. You are at the center of the square, and lines of energy crisscross each other and go through you. Energy moves horizontally back and forth, cutting through all parts of your body.
2. Visualize this energy as golden particles of light. Be in the center of this cube, and see golden light go back and forth and back and forth.
3. Breathe deeply, focusing on your feet. You don't have to do anything. Just bring your attention to your feet.
4. Now we will make a sound. When you make this sound, the energy

will crisscross much faster. This sound must be done quickly but not too fast: "Vami, vami, ma. Doot. Itoh mi. Sansha puri ryo. Zeme (zem-aaa). Zeme." Say the zeme set three times. "Zeme" is a very powerful word: "Zeme. Zeme. Zeme. Zeme. Zeme. Zeme."

5. When you make this sound, visualize the number 144. See this number on top of your head in a shining silver color.

6. This number (144) appears vertically, 1 on top, the 4 under the 1, and then 4 below the 4. Now chant: "Zeme. Zeme. Zeme. Zeme. Zeme. Zeme."

7. Millions of platinum 144 numbers pour into you. The 1 stands between your face and your crown, the 4 stands between your solar plexus and just above your heart, and the other 4 stands above your ankles: "Zeme. Zeme. Zeme. Zeme. Zeme. Zeme."

8. All the 144s are spinning now. Say, "Zeme. Zeme. Zeme. Zeme. Zeme. Zeme."

9. The 144s are breaking up and throwing a silver splatter of energy, and this energy goes throughout your being and your auric field.

10. Open your hands, and visualize 144 appearing in the middle of your palms. Turn both hands to a horizontal position [in relation to your body], and then turn them to a vertical position [in relation to your body]. Breathe. "Zeme. Zeme. Zeme. Zeme. Zeme. Zeme." Your hands might tingle, and you could feel some warmth, energy, or a tickle.

11. Now bring your palms to your heart, and lay them on your chest. Make the statement: "I am the energy of oneness."

12. Every cell recognizes the energy of oneness within you: "Every cell recognizes the energy of this oneness within me."

13. Here's one more thing you have to say: "I have become one with the One."

14. Bring your hands down now, and just breathe it in. Just take it in for a moment. Breathe it in. Now slowly open your eyes.

I feel different from when we started this. There is an expanded awareness of more than what is here on the physical plane.

This is called joining together, connecting you with you.

So this is joining with interdimensional aspects of my consciousness. Is that accurate?

Yes. You can even have a new name if you would like. This is called joining with the quantum body consciousness. You can definitely feel the energy shift in this.

Yes, I do. My sense is that the physical is here, but there's something else beyond a veil. That's kind of my sense of it.

It is true. Yes. This means you are not only integrating the energy of your quantum body but also starting to live from this quantum body once you fully integrate it into your physical body. That means you will start having quantum experiences.

When you wake up in the morning, it is also good to say, "I am a quantum being, and I create and experience quantum experiences today."

That's beautiful. In other words, what I do here affects ...

Your other bodies, your other realities.

Other dimensions, yeah, I hear that.

In many other realities, you are in a higher consciousness, and when you start integrating your realities, you will be able to bring higher consciousness from that reality into your present reality, creating more peace and more of everything positive in life.

As well as draw on whatever those realities have to offer.

Of course — the qualities, the talents, the gifts, the abundance, and everything else. How do you know you are integrating energy? When you are in a deep state of relaxation or meditation, you might hear some whispers, a soft voice, or singing, and you will say, "Who is making that sound?" There is no one behind you; it is you. You are experiencing you in another reality.

You could be sitting and suddenly feel a touch, and you say, "Who is in the room?" Nobody is in the room. It is a higher part of you. This exercise could be done every day, and we recommend doing it for a minimum of 21 days. After the meditation is finished, we recommend that you sit in the energy of 144 for 9 to 12 minutes. Sit in stillness visualizing 144.

When you do this, sometimes you will feel that you are carrying some energy in the front of your body because you will have 1 with you, 4 in the middle of your body, and another 4 at the ankles because you are carrying more of yourself. You'll always feel, "I am carrying more of myself. I am more grounded. I carry more of me — new ideas and more abundance. I'm carrying with me now more and more of myself." It's very, very beautiful.

It is. It is beautiful. I can kind of feel ... I'm getting inklings of this now, but it's not, obviously, just impressions.

This is the sound you must keep chanting slowly when the number 144 opens up. This is like a mantra you keep on chanting. This is a galactic sound from the planet Arcturus. Close your eyes for a moment, and say it with full feeling: "Zeme."

Zeme. Zeme.

In your mind's eye, imagine 144. "Zeme."

Zeme.

"Zeme."

Zeme. It's very powerful.

You will feel 144. "Zeme."

It resonates in my heart.

This sound is directly connected to your merkabah. You will see 144 take the shapes of a merkabah. "Zeme. Zeme. Zeme." You are in very good spirits, and when the merkabah comes, you are ready to fly.

Would you define what a merkabah is?

You can call it the light vehicle for your travels. You will see shapes, and many times, you will see a merkabah filled with colors. You will see writing on the merkabah, which could be in the ancient text of the Hebrew letters.

Does the Hebrew language originate off the planet?

The Hebrew language is a galactic language that was given to human beings with the permission of Lord Melchizedek. The frequencies of many of its sounds are quite powerful. They evoke certain emotions beyond the physical body that also awaken feelings and understandings.

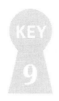

Open to
Receive Light

The Family of God

Family of God: Hello, my brother. We are the Family of God, and our love surrounds you. Now we are ready to start ascension key 9. We understand that ascension key 8 touched you deeply — the number 144 and the tone.

Yes.

Key 9 is about opening up to receive. This starts with a simple meditation to open you to higher consciousness and to access more of your soul's energy, vision, wisdom, and experience. This is an exercise we wish you to participate in, my brother.

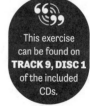

This exercise can be found on **TRACK 9, DISC 1** of the included CDs.

1. Imagine a golden ship the size of a vase. See it oscillate back and forth, as a ship rocks at sea, to the left and right, to the left and right. It is centered at your navel. Sometimes it goes very high, moving up to your shoulder, and sometimes all the way to your head.

2. When the ship goes up, see it being grabbed by hands of light, taking it upward and then spinning it downward, making a circle around your head. Now it moves to the top of your head and then

spirals downward, making a circle around your head. Be in this space.

3. See a light coming through an opening on top of your head. It shines out like a perfect ray of light. Both sides of this passage are lined with the magenta lotuses leading up to a small temple.

4. There are lamps on the walls of the temple and a small lamp on the top of the temple. As you enter the temple, you see it is a temple of receiving. The name of this temple is Numryo Temple.

5. The priest of this temple comes forward. His name is Ardhana, and he gives you a golden plate. You take it. The plate has a lamp in it. You hold this golden plate in your hands.

6. The lamp goes into your heart. You chant these words: "Sahi [sahee], sahi, sahi, sahi, re ma [rayma], le va ii [lee va eye]. Sahi, sahi, re ma, le va ii. Sahi, sahi, re ma, le va ii."

7. See a goddess come toward you. She is the goddess of ascension, the feminine counterpart of Archangel Metatron. Her name is Samsu Ra Vi. She holds a golden bowl, and she pours liquid ascension light into your hands. Visualize that you are catching this light as she pours it into your hands, the liquid light of ascension. Feel this light. Drink from this light. This light is your life.

8. All the fingers of your left hand are closed in a fist except the index finger, which you hold vertically in front of your heart. The fingers of your right hand are also closed in a fist except the index finger, and that finger is held horizontally in front of your heart [figure 9.1].

9. Just stay in this space. "Oshu ya wa. Oshu ya wa. Oshu ya wa. Oshu ya wa. Oshu ya wa. Oshu ya wa." This means: "I Am That I Am. I am the light of God."

10. See the liquid light that has been poured into you fill you up. You are full of the liquid light. The goddess of ascension moves behind you and touches your shoulders, fully opening the chakras of the alpha and the omega. This is called raising the angel wings within you. Breathe it in. Tone: "Oshu ya wa. Oshu ya wa. Oshu ya wa. Oshu ya wa."

11. You might see many beings coming toward you. These are your guides and your angelic support beings. They come to honor you in this special ceremony. You are ready to receive your light, the

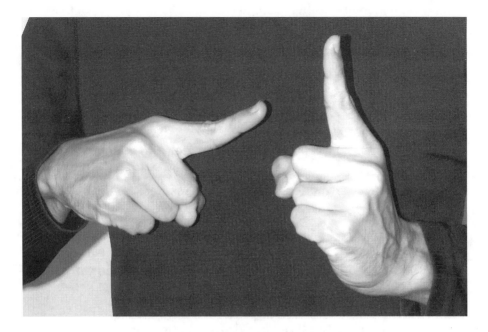

Figure 9.1. Mudra to open to receive light

light poured by the ascension goddess. You now accept this light and receive it, for now you know: "I am a worthy being, worthy to receive the light of God within me. I am the light." Tone: "Oshu ya wa. Oshu ya wa. Oshu ya wa."

12. Be in this space for a few moments while holding this mudra. The light from the goddess belongs to you. You see a flame in your heart, burning softly but brightly. It is a beautiful white. Be in the warmth of this flame. This is who you are — a flame of light, a flame from God.

13. Breathe the light in three times. Breathe it in. Breathe it in. Breathe it in. You may slowly open your eyes now.

How are you now, my brother?

It is hard to put it into words, but I could feel some of what was happening. It's like being touched on a very deep level that I have not experienced before.

Yes. We suggest that people who have difficulty in receiving do this exercise for 21 days. They will receive many other things, not just the light.

Call for Master Ardhana

Do the mudra from the previous exercise [figure 9.1]. Call on Master Ardhana nine times, and you might feel a sensation in your heart area. An opening might happen. "Ardhana. Ardhana. Ardhana. Ardhana. Ardhana. Ardhana. Ardhana. Ardhana. Ardhana."

My heart is opening up amazingly.

A passageway is created in this space, and Master Ardhana appears. He looks like a Buddhist monk. He is bald, and he wears a white robe and has wooden beads around his neck. He is quite muscular and healthy. He looks as if he is between thirty and forty years old, but he is thousands of years old.

Whenever you need to connect with your light, you can call Master Ardhana to lead you to the temple of light. Then when you call the goddess — "Samsu Ra Vi, Samsu Ra Vi" — you might feel a little pain in your heart area. This pain happens because at a deep level, you still resist your light. You still believe deep, deep down that you are not worthy to receive the light, so there might be some discomfort in the heart. Say, "Samsu Ra Vi, Samsu Ra Vi. I call to the goddess of ascension, Samsu Ra Vi."

See the goddess come to you. She is very tall. You can tell right away that she does not belong to this planet. Say, "Samsu Ra Vi."

I can feel the effectiveness of it for sure.

So this is the meaning of receiving. When you integrate the energy of receiving light, you say, "I am ready to receive all other things related to the light," because there is nothing that is not light. This ensures abundance in every aspect of your life. Your life will shift because now you are ready to receive everything. Everything is light at this level.

Become One with the Universe

Now we would like to show you a mudra and give you some more tones. You can tone the sound when you do the mudra. Make the mudra [see figure 9.2]: The thumb and index fingers of the left hand touch, and the other fingers are splayed, forming an "okay" sign. All the fingers are closed on the right hand except the index finger, which points upward. The right thumb touches the left palm with the closed fingers fitting over the left index finger. Both hands are held at the

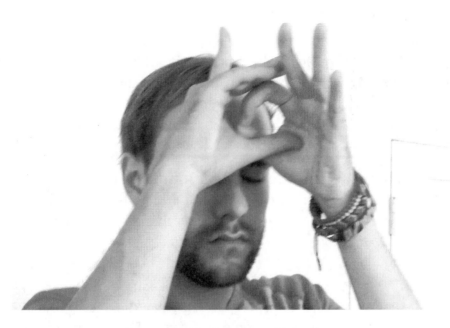

Figure 9.2. Mudra to become one with the universe

forehead in front of the third eye. In a matter of a few seconds, you will become still and one with the universe. Tone the sounds "oshu ya wa. Oshu ya wa." You might see galaxies and other realities open up.

My heart is definitely opening up to this.

This means, "I am one with the light. I am one with the universe." Slowly you will become a star. You are one of the stars in the universe: "oshu ya wa."

What I feel is a sense of belonging there.

You are the bright star in the universe. "Oshu ya wa. Oshu ya wa." This toning might surprise you. It is one of the names used for Master Jesus in other realities: "oshu ya wa." When you tone this for a long time, you will see this master walk in your energy field as a huge being, perhaps 20 feet tall.

Oshu ya wa.

"Oshu ya wa. Oshu ya wa. Oshu ya wa. Oshu, oshu ya wa." Relax, and you might feel a lot of energy and tingling.

I do. It's quite amazing.

How do you feel, brother?

I feel very lifted.

So this is called receiving the light, and you will also feel the energy of every eternity. This means receiving the light and everything else that is part of the light. It is the same as saying, "I am worthy to receive the love of God within me, and I embrace this love. I accept it, and I become this." This, along with Master Jesus, will support you.

Ask Lord Melchizedek to Clear Impacted Emotions

The human body has organs, tissues, muscles, bones, and blood. Another reason you might not be able to receive is your muscles hold many energies.

Yes, probably emotions.

These energies have been embedded for eons — the energy of fear, the energy of lack, the energy of false ego, the energy of looking for validation from other people, and so on. These energies have become as solid as rock, so even when higher frequencies of light come in, you are so hardened that they are not able to penetrate this deep, dense energy held in the body. When you make a road, you might need a jackhammer to break through rock. These energies have become hardened over time. Many people meditate and bring in light, but they are not able to fully push the light into these tissues because of the hardness.

You can call on the master of the universe, Lord Melchizedek. "I call on the energy of Master Melchizedek to come to me. I am asking that Lord Melchizedek's energy enter my bones, tissues, muscles, organs, bloodstream, head, teeth, and skin — my entire physical reality, my physical body. I ask that all the dense energy be flushed out." When you do this, you will experience the difference, even in one day. The next morning or evening, you will see a difference. Light is trying to come in, but there is so much density in your physical body that the light cannot penetrate it.

This is Lord Melchizedek's specialty. You don't have to do anything. Just ask to meld energy between you and Lord Melchizedek. See the beautiful platinum light come into and go out of your heart, your ears, your eyes, your nose, your mouth, your tongue, your hair, and your rectum — every part of the body, every tissue and muscle, because each part of the body holds different frequencies and karmic energies from all your lifetimes.

For example, you had a belief system about something from your past, a belief that maybe someone has cursed you or your family. This was a very common thing in past lifetimes. You believed in the curse and felt that things were not going to be good for you because there was a curse on the family. This is held in the ankles of the body. The feeling of unworthiness, "I am not good enough for the world" — you feel overly criticized and fearful — is stored in the kidneys.

So let's go back to the curse. When people feel that they have been cursed, they can simply ask Lord Melchizedek for help to diffuse this energy as they focus on their ankles?

Yes, exactly. Every organ carries the frequencies and karmic energies from all lifetimes. So when you contact Lord Melchizedek, ask that your tissues, muscles, organs, blood, and bones be fully cleansed and purified, and ask for everything that needs to be released to be cleared so that you can become a vessel to receive the light of ascension.

You'll see the difference, brother. Do it in the morning for about 20 minutes, and you will feel an uplifting kind of excitement come to you.

It's simply a meditation? There's no mudra, just a simple request that you meditate on and receive?

Yes. You can ask Lord Melchizedek to channel energies into your navel because your navel contains many energies and emotions, as well as the rejection of several past lives. You have been told that you are no good and that you are not fit for anything. All kinds of rejections are embedded there. When you carry rejection, you seek validation from other people by being too nice, too giving, or too apologetic. You want validation. Human beings need validation, but spending your existence seeking validation is what we are talking about. And that is held in the navel area.

So ask Lord Melchizedek to bring the energy to shield you from rejection energies, and ask that all past rejections be released. The energy of rejection runs through many lifetimes and all realities. We encourage you to do this for three days, and you will see some differences. Simply ask the light to come, and then see a beautiful platinum light anchor into all parts of your body. Ask for each part specifically: organs, tissues, muscles, bones, blood, hair, nails, teeth, and so on. This will take 10 to 20 minutes. It is a very good exercise for cleansing. It will take you deeper and deeper.

Human beings have built prisons for themselves from their thought processes of what they believe has happened to them. When you do this exercise, the walls of the prison will fall, and you will be liberated.

Activate Your Inner Security

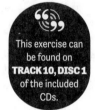

This exercise can be found on **TRACK 10, DISC 1** of the included CDs.

The next exercise is from Archangel Michael. There's a specific energy in your temples and above the third eye that must be activated. This energy is for inner security.

1. Close your eyes. Focus on both temples and just above your third eye. Imagine that connecting these spaces creates a triangle. Focus on this for 5 to 10 minutes.

2. Ask that the energy of inner security be activated. Say, "I ask to activate the energy of inner security right now." Breathe into this area. Focus on the triangle form created by connecting your temples and your third eye. Breathe into that area. Breathe.

3. You might see an opening on the top of the triangle. The triangle could be a light orange-red color or any color. Breathe into this triangle, and repeat this statement three times: "I am my inner security. I am my inner security. I am my inner security."

4. See these words line up inside the triangle. They are stacking up: "I am my inner security." The whole triangle is filled with these words as lines of energy.

5. There is an oil lamp at the top of the triangle. Inside the lamp, there is one word: "security."

6. See the word "security" go into your forehead horizontally. It is embedding there, imprinting security.

7. The word is repeated in a line that extends around your head creating a headband. Printed on the headband you can read "security, security, security." You are wearing the headband of security. It is silver.

8. The headband extends to form a beautiful cap shaped like a pyramid over your head.

9. This cap slowly sinks down into you. You grasp it, and slowly pull it down to your stomach area near your navel. You can see this cap there.

10. Every day when you wake up in the morning, bring your attention to your stomach and say, "I awaken my inner security cap and my inner security energy." Watch as an incredible light emanates from there, filling you.

11. Breathe it in. Slowly open your eyes now.

How are you now, brother?

I feel a lot of energy shifting. I can feel things are being adjusted and stuff is leaving. I am really being lifted.

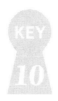

Assimilate the Feminine Energy

The Family of God

Family of God: All these goddesses have qualities that must be fully integrated for ascension energy. All are of galactic origin. You might call them extraterrestrial beings supporting humanity.

Goddess Aa Ri Ma:
Nurturance

The first feminine master you can call is a goddess from Arcturus. Her name is Aa Ri Ma. "Ma" means mother, referring to mother energy. "Aa Ri" represents the nurturing feminine aspect within you. This must be awakened and balanced with the other aspects of your life. A true mother is a nurturing mother.

Look at how animals love and nurture their young ones. They lick their fur and their eyes. They teach their young how to hunt. Nurturance is an integral aspect of feminine energy.

What does nurturance mean for a male human? It means being good to yourself. This is not ego fulfillment. Rather, this means nurturing yourself into the wholeness you are — nurturing yourself into your true self. When you awaken the nurturing aspect in you, you will start nurturing other people so that they can come into their power. Then you set them free.

Goddess Aa Ri Ma can support you in activating your ability to nurture. This is an integral part of ascension.

Goddess Kaa Rii Ma:
Hear and Understand Truth

The next goddess is Kaa Rii Ma. This goddess has a very special ability. She helps you hear and understand the truth, verify it within your heart, and then implement it. She is part of the Ashtar Command. She supports you to hear the truth on a very high level. For example, when you listen to music, you will enjoy it more. You will feel its richness. It will speak to you because you are hearing with your entire being. You will be able to capture the rich flavor coming from the sound frequencies.

As you ascend, it is very important to be able to hear and perceive the truth, filter it through your heart, compare it with your truth, and implement it in your life. Then you can experience it, share it, be with it, express it, and become it. This starts with hearing. Kaa Rii Ma supports the activation of this important quality.

Goddess Hea Ma:
Clear the Mind

The next goddess is Hea Ma. She is related or energetically connected to the goddess Pallas Athena. This goddess helps you clear your mind. Your mind constantly makes thought waves, sometimes unconsciously and sometimes consciously. When the mind is not still, it is not clear, and then it is difficult to perceive the truth. Even if the truth is being presented in front of you, you might not be able to comprehend it. Some people ridicule the truth. Look at the world now. How many people are willing to listen to the truth? Very few.

Clearing the mind is very important. Working with the energy of Hea Ma can support clearing the mind. Close your eyes, and say, "Hea Ma."

Hea Ma.

"Hea Ma. Hea Ma."

Hea Ma.

"Hea Ma."

Hea Ma.

Focus on the forehead, where your hairline meets the crown. "Hea Ma."

Hea Ma.

"Hea Ma."

Hea Ma.

"Hea Ma."

Hea Ma.

"Hea Ma."

Hea Ma.

This is a place called the truth chakra. You will feel a vibration, and you might even see spaceships or galaxies. "Hea Ma."

Hea Ma.

"Hea Ma."

Hea Ma.

"Hea Ma."

I can definitely feel the energy there.

Exactly. When your truth chakra opens, you will perceive the reality of higher consciousness, and you will accept it. The problem for most people is even when truth is presented to them, they cannot accept it. Their bodies are not clear. If a PhD-level textbook is given to a small child, the child will not understand it. She might tear out a page and make an airplane.

Goddess Hea Ma can support you to accept the truth. It will become so clear that every fiber of your being will say, "This is my truth." When you hear truth, you will not have to confirm it with anyone. It will awaken your wisdom, and you will just know it. Hea Ma can help you come to this place in every moment of your life. You will stand in truth all the time.

When you have truth and wisdom, these are your sword and shield as you walk this planet. You will have great courage. Truth will always set you free.

Goddess Ai Hi:
Plant the Seeds for Righteous Living

The next goddess is Ai Hi. This goddess plants the seeds for righteous living. She plants the seeds for a good crop to be harvested. When you plant a seed, it needs many things — sunshine, nutrition from the ground, the support of the elementals, love, and nurturance — so it can emerge as a small plant that becomes a tree, which bears fruit. Ai Hi helps you plant a seed for righteous living.

Here is something to remember: When you start down your ascension path, you must observe your life and take serious steps. How can you move through your life? Which things do you need to work on? Which things do you need to let go of? Where should you plant seeds? Where do you have patterns and behaviors? There are many factors. Self-improvement work is very critical for ascension. Part of this process is purification. Ai Hi helps you to plant the seeds of righteous living.

We will give examples of how to call on the goddesses at the end of the chapter.

Goddess Annho Ma:
Maintain Energy Levels

The next goddess is Annho Ma. She is part of the Ashtar Command. Annho Ma helps you connect with plants, minerals, crystals, and stones. These elements are part of your reality. Annho Ma also helps you create breathing patterns that can sustain your highly evolved energy. Even if you can raise your frequency, you might not be able to sustain it over long periods. Annho Ma maintains the frequency. She helps you understand breathing patterns and how to hold the frequency of the energy you have raised.

It is very important to sustain your raised frequency because the effect is cumulative. The energy you gather tomorrow is added to energy that you gathered today. It is not depleted. This is a big problem for humanity. When you are in a meditative state, you create good energy but do not sustain it. For most people, it drops considerably. This goddess can help you sustain your energy level today and then add to it tomorrow.

You must continue to increase your light without losing what you gained. Annho Ma helps you with this.

Goddess Za Ha Ma:
Understand Timelines

The goddess Za Ha Ma helps you understand the crisscross of different timelines. Timelines bring the experiences you need to overcome, learn from, and release. For example, suppose your life is going very well. Everything is good. Suddenly something happens. You wonder how you created this situation. This means a timeline crisscrossed, with your soul's permission, to bring an experience to your life.

This could happen for three reasons: to balance the energy, gain wisdom from the experience, or reveal the need to release an experience. This is very important. It is something that most people are not aware of. Lightworkers pray, meditate, and feel the energies from the other side, and still they have challenges and tests. They might think that they are doing everything correctly and wonder why they have challenges and tests.

Anchoring higher light and experiencing tests and challenges are two different things. You have the tests and challenges to balance the energy, gain wisdom, or release experiences. The goddess Za Ha Ma can help you to understand.

Goddess Pa La Ma:
Understand Your Blueprint

The next goddess is Pa La Ma. She helps you to understand the purpose of your life in your culture and your gender. Perhaps you have a bodily dysfunction. Pa La Ma shows you how to redesign your blueprint.

Goddess Pa La Ma is located on the planet Venus and is associated with the great teacher Sanat Kumara. When you fully understand why you were born into your culture and accept your culture and your body, you can have peace in your heart. You will not look to change who you are. You will say, "There is a purpose for being here in this physical body, and I am going to accept this part of me now." Pa La Ma can help you with this.

Goddess Ve Pu Nn:
Control Ancient Remembrances

The next goddess is Ve Pu Nn. She represents ancient civilizations and your ancientness on Earth. She is associated with the chakra in the space between your knees. It is connected to all the lives you had in the ancient civilizations of Earth. They are very old.

This chakra is actually not attached to the body. It is an energy that exists between the knees. Is that correct?

Exactly. This goddess helps you to understand your ancientness. When you understand your ancientness, you can open to wisdom. You are able to remember. Wisdom comes through remembrances. You will be able to go back in time. This is now blocked because human beings would not be able to process and live their lives if they remembered everything. The brain has a certain capacity, but the body is not fully fit to remember everything. This could be damaging in a very big way.

Can you explain that more?

Yes. People who take drugs have visions, and many are not able to handle the energies.

It blows their minds.

Exactly. This is why. The mind is very powerful. You are talking about 5 billion years. Just imagine if all those memories came back to you. Would you be able to handle it, brother? I'm sure not. People are conditioned to certain things in certain ways because they would not be able to handle the totality of their experiences.

It is not necessary to remember everything, but there are some memories and energies you must have for the ascension process, and this goddess can help you have the experience you need for ascension at the right time. For example, you have had a challenging situation for many years and have worked hard to overcome it. This goddess can help you understand the cause and effect of that energy: What started this? She can take you back to the lifetime energy that needs to be cleared from that side, and this can affect the situation in this lifetime.

Goddess Ve Pu Nn also works with the energy of Saint Germain. The violet flame of Saint Germain, if used properly, can help you remember by clearing your energies.

Goddess Aa Pa Ra: the Office Manager

The next divine goddess is Aa Pa Ra. She helps create a pathway for you to follow, bringing all parts of you, all your wisdom, so that you can move forward. She is called the office manager.

Aa Pa Ra organizes everything and makes a presentation to the company's CEO so that the CEO can make a decision. This is a very important job because she has to be aware of everything needed for the higher good of the company. This goddess helps by bringing all the wisdom, understanding, and people together to create your pathway.

Goddess O Ri Ka La:
Creative Force of Sexual Energy

The next goddess is O Ri Ka La. She helps you understand the creativity that exists in your sexual energy. This is the energy of pure creation, and it can be utilized to create a higher reality. Human beings are always trying to create a better reality for themselves. All people want things in their lives to be better, but they do not understand the process of creation through which they can improve things.

How is a human being made? Humans came from sexual energy. That is the energy of creation. How can you use this energy to create a better life? This goddess can help you do that. This is a very important concept.

You were born through the energy of creation. When you are on a path of ascension, you increase your frequency. You must also be able to create what you need to sustain you. Creation becomes very important, whether it is just to sustain your simple needs or to have the grander things in life. It does not matter.

It is important to be able to sustain yourself with your creation energy, and this goddess can help you use that creative force within you. This energy exists in both males and females. She also works with Archangel Michael.

Goddess Isha Na:
Define and Experience Love

The next goddess is Isha Na. She helps you define and experience love. Love has been described in many ways. Some people call it a frequency. Some people call it a feeling. Some people call it a thought. Some people call it an action. All of these are parts of love, but there is a higher meaning for love.

Love means pure creation energy, and that is who we are. The Family of God is called Creator, and we are pure creative energy.

Goddess Ooo Ma Me:
Safety

The next goddess is Ooo Ma Me. She represents the goddess of safety. Safety is important because when you feel safe, you open up more. You become your natural self.

Small children feel safe in the company of their fathers and mothers, especially when their homes are very loving. Children are able to express themselves fully.

The animals in a loving home are very natural. Look at your cats. They sit on you, they sit on the sofa, and they climb because they feel very safe in your home.

Yes, they do.

They are very natural. They don't feel afraid. When you are not afraid, you will show more of yourself, and you will share more of yourself. People do not show or share themselves because they feel they could be victimized or taken advantage of. This comes from a closed heart.

This goddess can help you create safety. Her name sounds beautiful: "Ooo Ma Me. Ooo Ma Me. I call on the goddess Ooo Ma Me." You will feel a very light feeling. Do you want to try it, brother?

Ooo Ma Me. I experienced a surge of energy run right down through my solar plexus.

It's beautiful and very soft. It is nice. "Ooo Ma Me. Ooo Ma Me. Ooo Ma Me. Ooo Ma Me." If you do it for a few minutes, you will feel as if there's something moving above your head, like stars and galaxies, and you become one with it. "Ooo Ma Me. Ooo Ma Me. Ooo Ma Me." How do you feel, my precious brother of light?

Pretty good here. Yes.

Good.

Goddess Haa Mum Ma:
Courage

Haa Mum Ma is a goddess who carries the energy of courage and is connected with the Goddess Sekhmet.

Yes, that's the Egyptian lion-headed goddess. Does this goddess work through Sekhmet?

Yes, but this goddess is also many other goddesses around the world. In India, she is called Kali.

Right. Very interesting.

Goddess Saha Ma:
the Divine Mother

The goddess Saha Ma is connected to the Shakti, the feminine power, a counterpart of Lord Shiva. She is the divine mother.

"Saha Ma." Close your eyes, focus on your heart, and say, "I call on the divine mother, Saha Ma." Say this nine times, please.

I call on the divine mother, Saha Ma. Saha Ma. Saha Ma. Saha Ma. Saha Ma. Saha Ma. Saha Ma. Saha Ma. Saha Ma. My heart has just opened up amazingly. It just seems so radiant. That's a good word.

Sa Bi Rar Kao:
Goddess of Wisdom

The next goddess is Sa Bi Rar Kao. She is a goddess of wisdom. If you open your palms and say, "Sa Bi Rar Kao," immediately you will feel energy in your hands.

I do, right in the palms.

Exactly. "Sa Bi Rar Kao." You will feel some tingling or energy moving in the middle of your palms.

I do, yes.

"Sa Bi Rar Kao." Goddess of wisdom. Okay. Can you feel it, brother, in your hands?

Absolutely, yes.

How to Connect with the Goddesses

You can connect with any of these goddesses by calling the name we have given you. We would like you to experiment, my brother. Tone this sound while focusing on the middle of your forehead: "Ai Hi. Ai Hi."

Ai Hi. Ai Hi.

"I call on Ai Hi Ma. Ai Hi Ma."

I call on Ai Hi Ma.

"I call the goddess Ai Hi Ma."

I call the goddess Ai Hi Ma. I definitely feel the presence in my upper forehead, above the hairline.

Okay. We will do one more. "I call on the goddess Ka Ri."

I call on the goddess Ka Ri. Ka Ri.

"Ka Ri."

Ka Ri. It's a different energy.

Exactly.

It seems more nurturing to me.

We will do another. "I call on the goddess Saha Ma. Saha Ma."

I call on the goddess Saha Ma.

Say it a few more times. "Saha Ma."

Sa Ha Ma. It's a different energy.

Yes. Now say, "O Ri Ka La Ma. I call on the mother, O Ri Ka La Ma."

I call on the mother, O Ri Ka La Ma.

"O Ri Ka La Ma." Say it like two words. "I call on O Ri Ka La Ma."

O Ri Ka La Ma.

"Ka La. I call on the mother, O Ri Ka La Ma. O Ri Ka La Ma. O Ri Ka La Ma."

Each has very different qualities. That's what I'm feeling, and they're very powerful. They are very, very powerful beings.

You can feel that the energies are different.

Yes.

There are many goddesses you can work with, but working with these goddesses can help you elevate your consciousness, sustain your frequency, and then build on what you have already achieved. You won't have to start over. This is one of the problems we mentioned before. Many people start over every day. Although they have built something up, they have dropped it, so they have to restart it.

You will be able to sustain your energies and grow from these practices. Then you can add to it. You will grow much faster. It is like making a building. Every day you add more bricks, and the building gets higher and higher. Eventually, you create a roof. You are building a house of ascension every day. Maintaining the energy is very important, and these goddesses can support you.

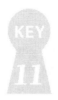

Activate Geometric Patterns

The Family of God

Family of God: Hello, dear brother of love. This is the Family of God. We are so honored to be working on this revelation of truth.

As am I.

Today, we discuss ascension key 11, which is a very extensive subject. It encompasses more than the geometric patterns in the body. When your light increases, this affects your chakras and the geometric patterns and codes within you — the spirit within your body and your beloved soul.

Today, we discuss the geometric patterns in the physical body. This subject has been reviewed by many people who have brought wonderful information. We will bring forth some additional understandings, and we encourage you to read about sacred geometry to gain greater clarity and wisdom.

Geometry is important because human beings are created through geometry. The sperm and the egg come together. Where did the egg and the sperm come from? They came from within you, from the very core of you, your spirit and your essence. You could simply call it the fullness of your self. This is represented by a sacred geometric pattern: the circle. It has no beginning and no end. In truth, a human being is without a beginning and without an end as an endless expression of divine life in many creative forms. This is why it has been said, "I shall be that I shall be." You are continuous and forward moving.

The first geometric pattern in a physical body is a circle. This circle, this cell, splits in two. Multiplication takes form in the cells, and this is called the vesica piscis, two intersecting circles. When this happens, the light of the universe is encoded with the vesica piscis. This vesica piscis is in the heart and the solar plexus. It could also be called the basis of the Father/Mother God energy within you, the Shiva and the Shakti.

Other geometric patterns include the triangle, the oval, the sphere, the rectangle, the tetrahedron, the cube, the flower of life, the octahedron, the dodecahedron, the hexahedron, and the icosahedron. These geometric shapes have vibrational frequencies and masters associated with them. This means every person carries the energy of many masters in his or her sacred geometric patterns. You have often heard that a human being is a composite of many energies. These energies exist throughout your being, but a large majority exist in these shapes and patterns.

When you work with these sacred geometric patterns, you balance many aspects of yourself, including your chakras (the chakras will become naturally balanced when you work with geometric patterns), and you activate the energy of the masters associated with these patterns. These masters are vested with the responsibility of the sacred geometric pattern in the human body. When you connect with these patterns, you connect with the energy of the masters. The master embodies the main vibrational quality or essence.

The Circle

The circle is represented by Master Yeshua. It extends from your face up to the tenth chakra, 10 to 12 inches above your crown. Brother Robert, close your eyes and visualize a beautiful, white, two-dimensional circle above your top lip. It extends up to the tenth chakra. This white circle is filled with brilliant colors. Breathe into this. You might feel a little nauseous or as if your head is spinning. Just breathe into this.

I feel a little nauseous, nothing significant.

Exactly. We just want you to feel the energy now. If you would like to make it stronger, you can make the sound "aung, aung."

Aung, aung.

See the vibration of this sound move into the circle. You will feel the circle fill up with this sound. The sound will vibrate like coils of light inside the circle.

Yes. I can sense that.

"Aung, aung." Sometimes it also feels like many light bulbs going off inside the circle, each like a coil of light.

I feel that this is opening my heart as well.

Of course, everything is affected.

The Tetrahedron

You have a tetrahedron between your throat and your ribcage. This tetrahedron is connected to Archangel Gabriel, and it represents the universal light encoded within you. Visualize this tetrahedron as a pale green color, and make the sound "vuu, vuu." You will see this tetrahedron begin to vibrate.

Yes, I have that sense.

It oscillates on both sides. "Vuu, vuu." Again, there's a possibility that you could feel nauseous when doing this for a few minutes, and you might feel a pressure on your third eye.

The Cube

You have another sacred geometric pattern beneath your ribcage that extends to your solar plexus: the cube. It represents oneness of body, mind, and soul and the I Am presence. It also represents the ability to balance the elements within you. The masters who help you open the cube are Master Kuthumi and Master Saint Germain. Both these masters work diligently to change this planet's vibration. The sound for opening the cube is "anddar, anddar."

Anddar.

You will feel some fluctuation or a pulling in the heart, not pain, but a slight discomfort. This can happen when you make this sound:

"anddar." Sometimes it can take you to a dark place in your mind, taking you deeper into the dark place. It's like sinking into an abyss.

Anddar.

"Anddar." You might see an opening, a passage, and you go through this passage into the darkness. "Anddar, anddar, anddar."

I feel it more in my solar plexus.

Yes. Good, brother.

The Vesica Piscis

Beneath the cube, you have the vesica piscis, two intersecting circles. This place represents the energy of the two opposing polarities coming together, the perfect balance between two opposites. Mother Mary holds the vibrational frequency for this: love and fear, yin and yang, day and night, Sun and Moon, the balanced energy of the Father/Mother God. This is on your solar plexus. The sound is "waheet, waheet."

Waheet, waheet. I feel it on my solar plexus.

You might feel pain there. "Waheet, waheet." When you do this, you will be able to strengthen this part in your physical body. Your mind will become strong and determined, and you will have courage, faith, and trust in yourself. You will strongly believe in yourself. The energy changes and becomes softer and whiter.

The Flower of Life

The next geometric pattern is the flower of life. It is between the second and first chakras. It is represented by Master Melchizedek and Master Thoth. The sound for it is "zumm, zumm."

Zumm, zumm. It really activates that area amazingly.

Let's say it twelve times. Close your eyes. [Repeats "zumm" twelve times.]

Zumm, zumm. I feel that this is strengthening the second chakra. It is resonating there a lot.

Yes. You will see beautiful light emanating from that area.

The Octahedron

Beneath the flower of light, we have a beautiful shape called the octahedron. This extends between the first chakra and the top of the knees. This place is overseen by Archangel Metatron, representing the atoms of creation — how the universe was created using patterns — repeating endless patterns. He holds this frequency.

Now, brother, close your eyes and bring your attention there. Simply focus on this area. You can make this sound: "annrhi, annrhi."

Annrhi.

Repeat this six times.

Annrhi, annrhi, annrhi. Annrhi, annrhi, annrhi. It's amazing, you know?

Can you feel something moving there?

Yes, I can feel a lot of activity there. It's hard to describe it.

There is a really powerful energy there.

Yes, it feels powerful.

Simply visualizing this octahedron while meditating is a very powerful exercise.

The Dodecahedron

After the octahedron, we have the dodecahedron, which is at the back of the knees and extends down to the feet. The dodecahedron is overseen by the great teacher Master Hilarion. It represents the human body and the interactions it has with heaven and Earth. Focus your attention there, at the back of your knees all the way to your toes, and make the sound "kinn, kinn, kinn."

Kinn, kinn, kinn. It really vibrates my feet. Wow.

Exactly. Say it nine times, and just be with the sound.

[Chants "kinn" nine times.] My impression is that it makes this part of the body more powerful, so I can walk with confidence on Earth. Will people experience this differently?

Exactly. But most of them will experience energy.

The Crescent Moon

The next shape is the crescent moon. It is on the soles of the feet. This is the energy held by the goddess we call Lady Quan Yin. The crescent moon represents the ingredient needed to be able to function in life between heaven and Earth in a balanced way. That ingredient is love. If there is no love, there's nothing. Love holds everything together, and it is through love that you must walk Earth. That is why this energy is on the soles of your feet.

You must carry love and generate it. How do you do that? When you activate this energy, your steps anchor love into the very ground you walk. Make the sound "neyhaa, neyhaa, neyhaa." The "ha" should be a higher tone.

Neyhaa, neyhaa, neyhaa.

Focus your full attention on the soles of your feet. You might feel an energy go up into your feet in a corkscrew pattern. Or you might feel a warm sensation on the soles of your feet.

That's more what I'm feeling.

One very beautiful thing about these geometric patterns is that they are embedded in your physical body and your etheric body. Many of your physical organs carry heavy-duty karma from past lives. They are being healed, released, and transmuted by working with these geometric patterns, sounds, and higher frequencies of the masters.

The Hexahedron

The hexahedron is about 12 inches above the twelfth chakra, one arm's length above your crown. It is a beautiful platinum color. It is about the size of your skull. The master associated with this shape is Master Mahareya. He is one of the masters of the Family of God. As you focus on this area, you can make the sound "julm, julm, julm."

Julm, julm, julm.

You might feel as if light is showering on you, as if light rays are penetrating you.

My impression is that this is something I've never opened in this lifetime, and it seems very new, but it also, somehow, seems familiar. I don't know what that means.

It is very true. Up to this point, many people were not aware of this chakra. They were only aware of seven chakras. These are advanced tools for ascension, and they will seem familiar for people who have worked on ascension paths in other lifetimes. They will say, "I know this. I just know it in my heart."

Yes, it's like going into an old closet I haven't been in for a long time.

Exactly. "I remember this. I know this."

The Icosahedron

The next geometric shape is the icosahedron. It is about 1 foot behind the middle of the back of your body. It is the thirty-first chakra, opposite where the high heart is — behind you. The color is like a soft orange and beige swirl. Work with Master Abraham, and make the beautiful sound "taooo, taooo, taooo." You will immediately feel some sensation at the back of the body.

Taooo, taooo, taooo.

It can take you deeper and deeper.

I'm getting impressions of Egyptian temples, active ones, when they were working as mystery schools.

Beautiful, beautiful. Just continue for some time.

Taooo, taooo, taooo.

You will see Egyptian and Greek temples, and ancient memories will rise from when you walked in those places. The powerful spiritual experiences you had in those temples will open when you work with this. Sometimes your whole body will jerk and shake.

Taooo, taooo, taooo. There is also a sense of timelessness with this.

Exactly. You are going into the ancient past. Actually, you are going to your akash. You are going into places where you had great spiritual experiences in the past. Sometimes you will see that you were lifted into the skies of other planetary realities.

The Triangle

The next few patterns are part of your auric field. First, we have the triangle. There are many triangles embedded in your auric field. Imagine that you are sitting in a circle of triangles, and these triangles spin in clockwise circles around you. They have a life of their own. You hear these triangles making sounds. They're also downloading something into you. They can break into many small triangles and expand. How do you feel, brother?

Well, I'm not getting too much from this. I need some practice. There's no sound that we make with this?

No.

The Oval

The next pattern is also in the auric field. It is an oval. The oval represents the ability to understand the significance of your mother in your life. Your mother brought you life. She is as God bringing life to you. When you understand the significance of your mother, then you honor her.

We understand that not all mothers are benevolent, but during the time of birth, most mothers experience the Divine within them. It can be just for a split second, but they experience God birthing an aspect of God. Mothers are significant because without the mother, you could not have any of the experiences you are having in this lifetime and all your lifetimes.

Understanding and making peace with your mother is important, whether she has passed away or not. Simply honor her and thank her for birthing you through many lifetimes so that you can experience your trueness, your ascension, your *moksha*, your *samadhi*. Without her, you would not be here.

What are moksha and samadhi? I don't know those words.

They are ancient words from the Eastern tradition that describe the experience of enlightenment.

Is the oval in the body anywhere in particular?

No, these are all in the auric field.

The Rectangle

The rectangle is also in the auric field. It represents the base elements that are the main ingredients for all life forms. These are the base elements in a tree, a plant, an animal, or a human being. This means understanding and experiencing the base elements.

The Spiral

The last geometric pattern is a spiral. It is in your auric field about 12 inches in front of your third eye. Imagine this spiral, and breathe into it. You will see the spiral start breathing back to you as if it has a life of its own. A beautiful soft energy might move from your third eye in a spiral pattern and down into you. What's your impression, brother?

It's activating my third eye, for sure.

* * *

These are some of the geometric patterns in the human body and auric field. When you activate these patterns, you activate the energies inherent in these patterns. You build the foundation energy for all life.

Does this mean you have to meditate on these every day? No. Understand these geometric patterns — that this is who you are and that you are made of these patterns. That is called wisdom. When wisdom is awakened, your light naturally increases.

It is good to meditate on these shapes for some time. They are one component of the thirty-three keys. The wisdom of the universe is encoded in your physical body in geometric patterns.

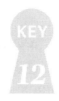

Embrace
Color Energy

The Family of God

Family of God: Hello, dear brother. We greet you in divine love and grace and hold you in the embrace of the Divine Father and Mother. Let us begin.

Ascension key 12 is about understanding the color spectrum in human physical and energy bodies. Human beings are fascinated by colors. The young, the old, the middle-aged: everyone is fascinated by colors. This world is made up of colors. They capture the imagination. They open different realities. They make you go within or take action. They make you contemplative or enter deep solitude.

Your color preferences change with age and time. A two-year-old girl might like the color pink. She wants pink dresses and dolls dressed in pink. When she grows up, her color preference might change. She might have needed pink at an early age to expand her ability to love and experience the energy of her heart.

Each color has a unique frequency and resonates with certain age groups. For example, some men wear pale-pink shirts. They choose this color unconsciously because it calls them to open their hearts.

In the past, this was not always culturally accepted. Some felt that men should not wear pink, that they should not open their hearts and show emotions. They should be the hunters, the warriors who defend the forts, fight the enemies, and slay dragons. They felt men were not supposed to show emotions. When men cried, they were seen as weak.

But now there is a pulling at the heart. You should open your heart because that is what is happening on the planet. Subconsciously, men are choosing pink — pink handkerchiefs or pale-pink shirts. There is some resistance, but there is still a pull, and men are going to follow the pull.

When you were in your mother's womb, you were engulfed in beautiful colors. The predominant color was gold, but other colors were associated with it. Pink was there, as was green, blue, white, and purple. These colors feed the baby's inner workings. Babies are nourished by their mothers and by colors.

Mothers are very aware of colors and how they affect the pregnancy and their emotional well-being. They choose colors for themselves, knowing that they support the babies they carry. When mothers understand color, they choose a spectrum of colors to support their babies to have balanced and well-rounded development of their personalities and emotional and mental bodies.

Wear Brown to Connect with the Earth

Very few people use the color brown, especially earth brown.

There was a time when browns were very popular but not now. In the 1920s and 1930s, they were very popular.

Earth brown is a very good color because it helps you connect with the earth. Early Native Americans had many earth colors in their garments, both men and women. They were much more connected to the land than people are now. This color must be brought back again so that people can be more grounded. When you are grounded, you are much more balanced and can fully embrace the present-day world, focusing beyond yourself rather than on what is going on around you. Soft brown can be a very powerful tool.

In the 1950s, 1960s, and 1970s, people used to wear earth brown shoes, but they don't wear them now as much. They wear different colors with a little bit of brown; they do not dress fully in brown. It is considered an old color. But this color supports you to come back into your reality and be a grounded person.

Leaves have a very big influence on your emotional body. Your internal organs also need specific colors to vibrate at their maximum capacity. Many colors feed your internal mechanisms.

All Life Emits Color

When you stand in front of a great painting, sometimes you feel touched. You want to stand and stare at this painting. Your internal organs can come fully alive. They suck energy from the painting because they do not have these colors within them. The organs "drink" the colors, and you feel good. You might reflect, "This painting is so beautiful. It speaks to me." What is really happening is the organs of your body are deficient in these colors, and they rebalance their frequencies so that they can function better.

Music also has color frequencies. When you hear beautiful music — great operas or classical music — you are not only affected by the sound of the instruments. The combined instrumental sound of an orchestra creates a spectrum of colors. These colors go into you. You are engulfed in a bubble of colors, and this affects your senses. You become drawn into the music. You hear the music, and you drink the colors.

You might say, "What amazing music! It is creating colors." Not all music produces beautiful colors. Some music produces unpleasant or repulsive colors. Beautiful music that touches your heart produces very soothing colors.

The Nutcracker is a beautiful ballet. The movement of bodies and the orchestral music send out colors. The audience becomes mesmerized. The colors and music affect the entire body. People watch the performance with their eyes, but the colors go through the entire body.

Mountains also emit energy and color frequencies. This is why there are often forests and vegetation on mountains. Mountains support the vegetation by sending out color frequencies suitable for that forest.

The animals also emit energetic colors. When they sing, they emit sound frequencies, which create color spectrums. Animals know this. As lions, cheetahs, or panthers look at their prey, they sense the energy of the animal, and they perceive the colors they send out. A cheetah picks up the scent, the essence, and the colors. It knows whether it should approach this animal or not. It does not attack all animals. It knows whether they can bring this animal down. Wild buffalo send out a color spectrum that says, "Don't come near us."

People do not understand the frequencies they emit. Brother Robert, how would you rate your sound? Do you think there's a color to the sound you emit?

Do you mean through my voice?

Yes, brother.

It would only be a guess. I have no idea.

You want to be aware of it. There is a color spectrum every time you open your mouth. Before your ear hears something, your body absorbs the sound frequency coming from someone's mouth. It happens in a nanosecond. Your body tunes in to the frequency of the colors emitted by a human voice and then absorbs the sound.

Experiment with it. You will be amazed. There will come a time when cameras or instruments capture the sound colors coming from a human voice.

When you die, you make a spectrum of colors. Your merkabah is used by your soul to travel, and it has colors inside it.

Each master has a specific color combination and frequency. Archangel Michael is blue. Archangel Metatron is platinum. Lord Buddha is golden. Quan Yin is orange-red. Lady Nada is green. Saint Germain is purple. Master Yeshua is brilliant white. When you call a master, close your eyes, and you will see his or her color fill you.

Revel in the Ocean's Beauty

Ocean waves emit seven frequencies of color. This is why most people feel good near the ocean, especially when few people are around and the waves are gentle.

How can we see the colors? Do we close our eyes and see them with our inner vision?

You will not see them, but you will be able to feel them with your inner vision.

We cannot see them physically?

You will when you offer more and more of yourself. Then you will be able to see more inner things with your eyes.

One of the colors emitted from waves is turquoise. This color is directed from your heart. Waves also emit light green. This affects your belly. They emit a beautiful soft pink that affects the throat. This is one reason people see beauty in their loved ones at the beach. The ocean tells them to express their feelings. They are in a safe place to let go. There is much love at the beach!

The ocean emits purple and gold. These colors flow above your head and down your back. They make you feel good, at one with nature.

Would it be accurate to say that at the beach, the crashing waves emit an energy of these different colors?

Yes, exactly, you got it.

So you feel the energy, and you can feel or sense the colors.

One day you will draw these colors. The next time you go, take your divining rods with you. We would like you to test it out.

The ocean waves also emit a soft indigo. This color massages your internal organs. Everything feels so relaxed because it releases all your worries and stress.

The ocean also emits a soft beige. This helps you develop new ideas. Next time you are stumped for an answer, go to the beach and visualize this color. Then ask the ocean, "Can you give me an answer to what I'm seeking?"

Connect with the Colors You Need

How can you perceive your individual color? You are aligned with certain colors during different periods of your life.

So color shifts as a person grows?

Exactly. When starting work after graduation, many men choose to wear blue suits, often with a white shirt and a red tie. When they are about forty-five years old, the colors of their ties and shirts might change. When they get older, the colors change again. The previous colors don't support them any longer.

How do you find your aligned color? There is a palette of colors in your medulla oblongata, in the back of your brain. There are eight colors embedded in this very important place. This is also what we call the storehouse of wisdom, light, and magic. These colors will not usually come to the forefront of your mind. But you can call on them to come into your life.

For example, suppose you need courage and determination. You are going to take action. You might call on the color red from your medulla oblongata. Now close your eyes. We will try an experiment.

Focus your attention on your medulla. Visualize a horizontal box with eight colors in it. Choose the color red because you want to have courage, determination, and action in your life. Breathe into this color, and pull it out through the middle of your forehead. Then hold your breath, and take it down to the soles of your feet and anchor it there. Breathe and connect with the red again.

You might feel some energy or pressure on your forehead. How do you feel, brother?

I feel fine. I can see the red. I'm not feeling anything associated with it at this point.

Okay. Let's say it's evening, and you are tired. There are many things on your mind, and you are not able to sleep. Going into the palette of colors in your medulla, pull turquoise forward. Breathe into the turquoise. Pull it out through the middle of the forehead, and take it all the way down and spread it on the soles of your feet. Keep breathing. Take about six breaths.

It's very relaxing.

You will see that in a few minutes your head and shoulders will relax. Suppose you are getting ready to go to a big meeting. You are full of energy and enthusiasm. You feel very confident. This is an important meeting, and you are going to meet a very important person. You want to be at your best. Inhale the colors beautiful metallic blue combined with gold. Inhale this nine times. See these colors go from the middle of your forehead and down to spread on the bottoms of your feet.

I can feel this and see it. What I'm feeling is confidence.

Exactly. This is what happens. You feel good.

The next color is white. Inhale the color white. Take it through your forehead, and spread it on both soles of your feet. Breathe it six times. Do you feel something, brother?

No. I can feel the white, but I'm not associating it with a feeling.

It simply means, "I am going to take a break. The world can go on, but I am going to take a break, relax, or sleep."

Maybe I'm not very good at that. I need more of that.

Sometimes you busily go through your lives and rarely take a break because you have to get so many things done. Inhale the color white, and think, "Let the world go on. I'm going to take a break."

The next color is beautiful magenta. Breathe into the magenta. From the forehead, spread it all around your ankles and feet. We will breathe this nine times. This calls forth the ability to see the larger truth or a higher position.

I got the magenta, but again it was hard for me to associate this with a particular feeling. Now that I know what to look for, I think that will help.

Also, do the last one. It is called "foccachio."

What color is that?

It is a combination of pink and orange.

Is it similar to coral?

A little bit darker than coral.

Okay.

Breathe into it. Bring it into both hands in the middle of your palms. You might feel some tingling in your arms.

I feel the tingling. I got the color. I'm guessing here, but I think it has to do with taking action.

Exactly, brother, you got it. Create the action. Once you understand that you have the color in your medulla oblongata, you can choose from these eight colors for whatever situation you want to empower or create. Work with them. For example, when you want to meditate, you can call on all these colors. If you want to take action, you can call one color and breathe into it. If you want to relax, you can call another color. If you want to understand something from a perspective higher than what you are reading in the news, call a color. If you want to feel confident, focus on another color. This becomes a tool.

When your ascension process really starts moving, many masters will continually work with you. You will know they have come into your presence because of the colors they emit.

Here is an experiment for you. Suppose you are going grocery shopping and you hear a child cry. A color is emitted when the child cries, especially if the child is fearful, so the crying is a shrieking sound. People often say this sound pierces their ears.

It is very irritating. It irritates many people. It irritates me.

The color sent by the screaming affects your auric field, and your aura reacts to it. When there is violence, a color is exhibited. This color is often dark black, and it repulses people.

Everything in the universe is moving. When something is being created, there is action, and there is a color associated with it. There is a color associated with lovemaking, especially when both parties have a true heart connection and join the body, mind, and soul. There is sacredness, honoring, and mutual respect. A beautiful color comes through both of them.

What is that color?

The colors of the rainbow.

Oh, so it's all colors.

Look at some of Alex Grey's paintings.[1] He paints the energy and the colors emitted when two people make love.

When a mother breastfeeds her baby with the purest intention, energy is sent out from her to her baby and from the baby back to her. From this, beautiful colors are created. Alex Grey is able to capture the essence of energy and the essence of the colors behind the energy.

Color is part of every energy field. Vegetables have different colors because they hold certain energies. Your body parts have colors associated with them. You will not be able to recognize them, but inside you have color codes. The main colors are in the pallet of the medulla oblongata. We do not encourage you to say that this is "my" color. You must be balanced in all these colors.

We call this place a storehouse of colors, frequencies, geometric patterns, and sounds. We are trying to bring you some understanding about the color, and we deal with geometry too. You will see how they blend to make a human being. Once you understand it, you don't have to focus too much on it, but this understanding will give you a higher perception of the energy you are taking on.

---

1.   View Alex Grey's works at https://www.alexgrey.com/.

You will be able to maintain a higher energy frequency. Just to give you some advice, a room that is painted orange is very stimulating and powerful. You don't often see the color orange in hospitals. Colors will draw out your inherent qualities. If the colors are too weak, people can become lethargic. You must balance things.

Many people choose neutral colors for their houses — off-whites.

But there are some orange offices. This is to keep pressure on people.

So someone who is seeking enlightenment or ascension must learn to master colors?

Yes. Once you become aware of colors and focus on them for 3 or 4 days, they will become a part of you. You don't have to work on individual colors. You can work on all colors in one sitting for 20 minutes.

That makes good sense. You're basically opening up the pathways in your consciousness to these colors?

Exactly. Enlightenment is a shift in the human mind. The shift happens because the brain becomes filled with beautiful manna, which is called the food of the soul. It is a beautiful platinum color.

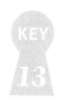

Anchor the Balance from Rainbows

The Family of God

Family of God: Hello, blessed brother of light. We are the Family of God. It's always an honor to connect with you, for you hold light. Remember that you are the light. We send our light into your light, adding more light to you.

Today we will talk about ascension key 13, the importance of the rainbow. Almost all people love rainbows. When a rainbow appears, people experience feelings of liberation and joy. Rainbows often appear after a rainstorm. When you see a rainbow, something clears, and new magic appears in the sky. The ancient ones called rainbows the love of God appearing in the sky.

A rainbow has many functions. Recently you might have seen images of a double rainbow or triple rainbow. More triple rainbows will appear in the future. There are certain frequencies of light and energy in rainbows. In fact, there are three spirits associated with rainbows. They are called rainbow spirits. They do not have bodies; they are of luminous form. Their names are Mathrun, Yamanockh, and Skymoiore. Skymoiore is feminine energy, and Mathrun and Yamanockh are masculine.

These three beings emit the energy of balance, and this is why people feel joy when they see rainbows. They feel clearer. Some people break out in smiles. Some take photographs. People feel good in the presence of a rainbow, for they receive the energy of balance. It is beamed into them by the rainbow.

Mental conflicts arise when there is imbalance between the male and female. Everything has to be in harmony: the energies of the heart, the mind, the body, and the bloodstream. Everything has to be harmonized. These beings send energy of harmony and balance into you. When there is harmony between the male and female polarities, most of your energies will automatically balance. Your magnetics and electrical energies will come together to create new alchemical energies called liberation and freedom.

You can call these beings and work with them daily to anchor the energy of balance in your chakra column, extending all the way from your twelfth chakra (one arm's length above your head) to the earth-star chakra (8 inches below your feet). These three beings hold three color frequencies: soft copper, soft white, and gold. Bring these three colors into your chakras — download them and anchor them into your twelfth chakra — and bring them through your body into your earth-star chakra.

When you bring this energy into a chakra, see your chakra spinning. It is not just that the energy comes in your chakras. Make the intention that your chakras are spinning, and then the energy flows through like a stream of light into the chakra. The chakra spins and rotates continuously. See the chakras rotating faster and faster. Then it will expel imbalanced energies, and your chakras will slowly take the shape of a big spindle. When you do this exercise with conscious intent, it can heal you and help you raise your frequency greatly.

How do you raise your frequency? Bring higher light into yourself, and clear the pathways within you to hold more of this light. Otherwise, even if higher light is able to come into your body, you are holding on to old emotions that don't support you, and there is no space for the new energy. Rainbow energy clears the pathways and creates openings for higher energy to enter and stay.

Use Rainbow Frequency for Awareness

Rainbows also have a sound frequency. This sound frequency is very simple. It is a musical scale — do, re, mi, fa, so, and so forth. When you visualize and call for the sound frequency of a rainbow, simply sing a frequency or series of notes. Repeat the notes and see them go into each chakra. A musical code will slowly emit through your voice, creating your individualized tonal frequency. This tonal frequency is your source voice. When toned, it will instantly bring you to a place of more conscious awareness. It is like a string that pulls you back into your core self.

There are many instinctive energies in your base chakra: survival, fear, fight or flight, manipulation, disruption, and other energies. But your base chakra also contains the energy of enlightenment, the kundalini.

Clear the Base Chakra

1. Visualize that your base chakra is a beautiful rainbow-colored pyramid. Focus on that and breathe.
2. You might see colors from the rainbow go upward in the shape of a tube, as if a string is attached to the rainbow pyramid and it is pulling the colors up into your second, third, fourth, fifth, sixth, seventh, eighth, ninth, tenth, eleventh, and twelfth chakras.
3. There is another rainbow pyramid at your twelfth chakra. Its apex points downward. You are connecting one rainbow pyramid at the top to another rainbow pyramid at the bottom. Breathe into that.
4. You will see a spectrum of colors of light going from the bottom to the top and from the top to the bottom. When this is done with conscious intent, you will release many past energies held in your chakras, and your entire energy spectrum will be cleansed and puri-fied. This will also affect your auric field. Breathe into it, one rainbow pyramid on top and one rainbow pyramid at your base chakra.
5. See a beautiful infinity sign form between these rainbow pyramids. Breathe into this. You'll see an infinity symbol moving slowly — vibrating and spinning. Breathe into this as you are filled with the colors of the rainbow in an infinity wave.
6. Continue to breathe into the image, and you will see this infin-ity symbol multiply into three. One goes between the pyramids, another wraps around you, and then you are inside a rainbow infinity sign. Breathe into it. Breathe into it.

This exercise can be found on **TRACK 11, DISC 1** of the included CDs.

This exercise can help you release unwanted energies that you pick up from all sources — being in an environment where there are other people, a television set, a computer, or whatever. You will be able to maintain a higher frequency at all times.

The Mother-Father Rainbow Energies

Rainbows can help you heal childhood traumas such as your relationships with your mother and father. Hold this intention, and place it into the rainbow pyramid. This is all that is needed.

If you can recall the sound of falling rain when you meditate, then you are meditating with the sound of a rainbow. This can enhance your experience and open your ability to sense and perceive all the creatures living on this planet — frogs, butterflies, spiders, and everything else. You can awaken this gift of being able to connect with these beings at their level of consciousness. You can also use recordings played in the background when you do this visualization exercise. This exercise is best done in the mornings when you wake up and are ready to start your day.

Rainbows also have mother and father aspects. The mother aspect helps you open to the nurturing, compassionate qualities within you. The father aspect helps you come up with ideas and solutions to create a better environment for your life and others' lives.

Rainbows are a full circle, but you only see half the circle in your realm. One half has father rainbow energy, and the other half has mother rainbow energy. Connect these two aspects to anchor and awaken new ideas and new solutions combined with compassionate nurturance. A rainbow's energies are connected to clouds, rain, and the elements. All of these have a significant influence on your body and energy field. When you work with rainbows, many energies can be supported.

Did you know that you can capture the essence of a rainbow in a glass of water? The rainbow appears when you place a glass of water near a window in the sunshine. Call on the father and mother spirit of the rainbow and the three rainbow spirits (Mathrun, Yamanockh, and Skymoiore) to fill your glass of water with the essence of the rainbow. You will feel a difference when you sip this water.

You can invite the rainbow spirit into your bedroom so that there is harmony among those sleeping there. If lightworkers collectively called the rainbow spirit and anchored this energy in the beautiful country called America, do you think there would be a difference?

Rainbow energy soothes and touches people. It is like your grandmother holding you and saying, "I know you are hurt. Come to me. Let me embrace you. Be in my arms. Don't think of anything now. Just be in my presence. Let me embrace you with the warmth of my heart."

Maintain Your Frequency with Rainbow Energy

Some birds are closely aligned with the spirit of rainbows: the parakeet, the peacock, the hummingbird, and a few others. These birds know the timing of rainbows. There are codes emitted from a rainbow before it appears to Earth beings and animal spirits. The codes are directed toward the water that people drink — a lake or a river from which drinking water flows. The waves are nurtured when a rainbow appears. It sends the energy of nurturance into water because water, by its very nature, is nurturing. But because of pollution in the environment, it does not carry the life force it is intended to carry. Water that comes from a dam is very angry because it has been stopped. Yet rainbows nurture water so there is enough love and compassionate energy in the water.

Rainbows also send energy to people who are ready to pass on to the next level of their life dreams so that they can go gently. If you study this carefully over time, you might see a correlation between rainbows and people passing away. Within twenty-four hours after a rainbow appears, many people pass away much more gently because they have been touched by the spirit of a rainbow.

Rainbow energies are encoded in sacred geometrical patterns. One is called the sri yantra. When you go to some great structures, like places of worship, you feel very good because sacred geometric patterns contain the frequency of a rainbow. You feel a sense of peace when you go to sacred places.

Rainbows do not only happen when rains come. They support the evolution of humanity in ways that people do not know. All vegetables and fruit are supported by rainbows, giving them energy in a soft, gentle way, asking them to grow healthily so that human beings can consume them and get the nourishment they need. Rainbows support the trees.

There will come a time when rainbow energy will be incorporated in bringing children into the world through natural childbirth. Native American people sing to the rainbow spirit. You might want to research this and learn the songs to the spirits of the rainbow and the Moon. We encourage you to work with the rainbow spirit to keep your frequency higher to maintain a state of awareness.

Now we will take some questions from you, brother, if you have any.

I have one question. To do these exercises, such as the one with the glass of water, do you need to be in the presence of a rainbow, or can you simply summon the energy by asking for it?

Initially, you may want to be in the presence of a rainbow when it appears, but once you are able to work and integrate these energies, simply calling on the frequencies of these three beings and the father-mother energy of rainbows is all that is needed. You might want to try it out tomorrow morning.

It's unlikely we're going to have a rainbow tomorrow morning.

It doesn't matter. You can call on the energy, and you will feel the difference. You can do it. You will start to see double rainbows, triple rainbows, and maybe, once in a while, quadruple rainbows — four rainbows appearing simultaneously. These rainbows will have many colors, not the colors you are used to seeing. Rainbows can support you to program your dreams.

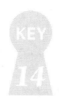

Download Dragon Ascension Energy

Dragon Spirits and the Family of God

Dragon Spirits: We, the dragon spirits, welcome everyone on the path to self-realization, self-acknowledgment, and self-love. These are important qualities. We have been on the Earth plane for billions of years not in physical form but as energetic forms. We were asked by the Council of Creators to come here to anchor our energy to support human beings when they come to Earth.

Some of the dragons' understanding has already been given to you. Brothers Rae and Robert have also done many workshops on dragons, and there is information on us in their books. [See appendix I, *DNA of the Spirit, Volume 1*.] Today, we would like to talk about ascension key 14, dragon ascension energy. Let us call forward the dragon Kinshihar.

Support for Cell Growth

Kinshihar: Hello, my friends. We are the rain dragon spirit. Our color is a beautiful metallic golden-green color. We do not breathe fire as shown in movies, comic books, or children's storybooks. We have a bigger role to play than to consume people with our fire. We are emissaries of light who have come here to push the planet in the right direction so that it has the potential to go where it needs to go. The rain dragon is very important because without rain, most species cannot survive. Rain is very important for human beings and for the planet.

We exist as part of your etheric body. We are way above your head, between the twelfth and the fifteenth chakras. Now, brother Robert, would you like to raise your hand one arm's length. This is the place of the twelfth chakra, the yamne chakra. We are between the twelfth and the fifteenth chakras.

So you exist in this place in the etheric bodies of all human beings? Is that correct?

Yes, and we are connected to the water of your physical body. You can live a long time without food, but you cannot live without water. Water is the essence of life. We are connected to water, and we are the beings who bring water into the physical body when a baby is in the womb. It is like magic how a life form is created, how a fetus takes on limbs and develops a body and a head. Do you call it magic?

Yes, I guess I do. It's inexplicable.

There has to be supportive energy for the original cell, and we are supportive energy. Let me give you an example. A bicycle is made in a factory, but there is something important that it needs in order to work — air in the tires. If there is no air, the bicycle will not move. In the same way, water is essential in a human body, and we supply water to every cell of a baby.

So the water you supply brings the magic of making a fetus or a body?

Exactly. You will be able to go back to that place in time when you were a single cell. This cell had full intelligence. It knew its goal. It had to find a receiving place where it could incubate and host life, so it had full intelligence. It knew where it needed to go. This can help you now. You need to know where you need to go. Human beings are lost. Many say, "I don't know where to go."

They don't remember who they are.

We know. Come to this cell, and it will know where it needs to go so that it can once again become the creative force, the inherent force, of this cell. It knows where it needs to go to incubate and produce a new life, and it knows where it needs to go to become a new you.

That's amazing. I guess you're going to tell us how to connect with that cell? Is that correct?

Just communicate with us. Simply say, "Kinshihar."

1. Close your eyes and imagine a beautiful golden-green light above the yamne chakra, the twelfth chakra.

2. Open your palms, and say, "Kinshihar." Say it in your own way.

This exercise can be found on **TRACK 12, DISC 1** of the included CDs.

3. Visualize the golden-green light coming to you. Chant "Kinshihar." You will feel energy all over your body, especially in your hands. You will feel the energy right away.

I do.

4. Chant "Kinshihar" nine times.

[Chants "Kinshihar" nine times.] What I feel is a sense of amazing benevolence and support.

Do you feel energy in your hands?

Yes, I feel that. I can see the color, the golden-green light.

5. Breathe in this color. Breathe it in, and imagine that you changed this energy into your pineal gland in the back of your medulla oblongata. You will see an explosion of light there.

I can feel the activity there in the medulla oblongata.

6. Exhale into the medulla oblongata nine times. Breathe and chant "Kinshihar" nine times, and exhale it into your medulla oblongata.

[Breathes and chants.]

How do you feel, brother?

My hands are tingling. I saw at one point a flash of white light in the pineal gland.

7. When a drop of water falls to the bottom of a bucket, there is a splash. You see a splash like that in the back of your brain. When this happens, it means the light is going into the pineal gland in which you hold your original cell. We call this the intelligent cell. It is also called the God cell, and when you are in touch with your God cell, you are able to make many changes. This is the place

where you were conceived, and the cell currently knows it came into full consciousness at the moment of conception.

That's amazing. It makes so much sense.

So join with us, Kinshihar. I will take my leave at this time, for our energy is very difficult for brother Rae to hold.

Trust in the Unseen

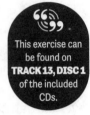

This exercise can be found on **TRACK 13, DISC 1** of the included CDs.

Family of God: The next dragon is Guruheva. This dragon helps to bridge the gap between the seen and the unseen. It is located in the etheric body under your feet. In simple terms, what this dragon does is help you to trust divinity and the divine plan in every moment of your life, knowing the higher purpose for every divine moment.

Guruheva: One of the main problems for human beings is they are always seeking proof. They want proof of things, but if they were to use the five basic senses, they would not seek proof. They would sense it and feel it.

As you review the history of the planet and study the scriptures of any religion, you see that people are told to have faith in the unseen. Don't ask for proof because this shows that you do not trust. It shows you have doubt. God can take any form. Scriptures preach about having faith in the unseen. You don't see the wind, but you certainly see the effect it has, don't you? It's like love. You feel love, but you do not see it.

We help people come to a place of being able to believe and trust in the unseen and in the various processes of life. So trust the process. People might say, "This process is very difficult. How can I trust?" You will come to a place where you can say, "I'm not doing everything. Everything is done through me. I am just a carrier of the action, and this action does not reflect who I am in my deep inner core." At that level, you will not have fear because you do not expect anything. You are just a carrier of actions, of the energy coming through you. You are just a doer, and you are not affected.

We support the integration of the energy of the unseen and the seen by helping you trust yourself. Your earth-star chakra extends from your feet. Our energy is about 20 inches beneath the earth-star chakra. When you start trusting, you will trust the higher aspects of yourself. You cannot experience your higher aspects unless you fully integrate and master your lower aspects. This means without Earth, you cannot experience heaven. You must fully join with the Earth spirit to experience the higher spirit.

It is very important to work with your first three chakras. Many traditions do not focus on the first three chakras, but this must be done.

1. Close your eyes. There is a tetrahedron, a sacred geometric pattern, about 20 inches below your feet. Breathe it in. The color of this tetrahedron is platinum.

2. Breathe it in, and you will see this tetrahedron start to move, and you will feel a tickle or a tingling on the bottoms of your feet.

I feel that. It goes up into my shins as well.

3. This tetrahedron will start to expand. Breathe it in. Breathe it in. It will come up to just beneath your feet. That means you are standing on the tetrahedron full of the platinum color. This is your magic carpet. You will feel as if you are floating or flying. The tetrahedron starts moving. It might scare you. It's moving you up, and you are floating. You are very connected to the ground, but there is freedom.

Yes, I can feel that. In a sense, it's like being freed from gravity.

Exactly, yet you are fully grounded.

Yes. I am very grounded.

4. But you are free from things. That means you are in the world and out of it. This is what Jesus taught. You are fully grounded on Earth, but you feel freedom in your heart.

Yes. It feels like mobility, like flying or something.

5. Exactly. And you will see beings appear. Sometimes you will see a roller coaster appear under your feet. You might be floating very happily, and suddenly you won't want to come down because you are floating, fully grounded with the earth. There is freedom there, and in that freedom, you begin to trust yourself and love yourself. That means you have bridged the gap between the unseen and the seen,

Now you know. Do you have any questions?

No. I am just experiencing this. It's pretty amazing. Like you said, there's magic here.

Release Fear

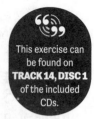

This exercise can be found on **TRACK 14, DISC 1** of the included CDs.

Arandataar: We are Arandataar. We are the dragons to release fear. We are connected to the threefold flame of your heart. We are closely associated with Master El Morya and the first ray of God. The first ray of God is called the Will of God. When fully activated, this ray helps your mind become focused. You become fearless, courageous, and incredibly powerful.

We exist in that etheric link, and we want to bring attention to your navel area and your second chakra area. Our color is copper. Our function is to release or remove distortions in your thinking, for we believe fear is created through your distorted thinking. If you think wisely, there is no fear, but if not controlled, distorted thinking can spiral downward. Is that not true?

It can get totally out of control.

Every human being goes through this problem at different levels.

1. There is a spiral between your navel and your second chakra. Visualize this spiral filling with a beautiful shining copper color. Breathe, and then what do you see? The spiral starts spinning and moving.
2. You see the spiral expand. Breathe, and let it expand. The spiral is rotating. It might rotate clockwise or counterclockwise. Breathe into that space, and see the spiral fill with a beautiful shining copper color. The spiral will extend outward.
3. Open your palms. The spiral extends to your palms and moves around your body. Breathe it in.
4. See this spiral in your hands. Put your hands together in prayer position in front of your body [figure 14.1]. Move them down to the area between your navel and your second chakra, fingers pointing away from you, and see the spiral move outward from your hands. It extends in front of you about 20 feet. Allow this, and then breathe it in.
5. You will feel a little spaced out, but continue doing this. Your eyes might blink. Your eyebrows might twitch. Continue doing this until you see sparkles of light and stars coming out of your hands.

I see the sparkles.

6. When that happens, release your fear. Extend your palms out in front of you. Allow the sparkles to move in their own way.

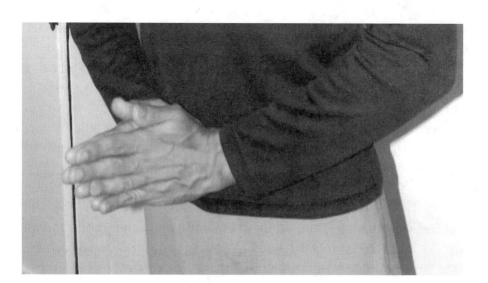

Figure 14.1. Mudra to release fear

The sparkles are all around. That's my sense of it, like stars all around me.

Exactly. Welcome this, and you will shed a lot of fear, anxiety, and insecurity in your life, the past actions that created fear in your life. You will see these shift. Your whole body will have a nice warm feeling.

I have the feeling of being comforted.

Yes, and you will feel like someone is embracing you or loving you and saying, "Hey, it's okay." You are in a very beautiful, relaxed space.

That's what it feels like.

Done over several days, this exercise will help you to relax. After working with this regularly for fewer than 30 days, 30 to 50 percent of your fears will leave — the fear of survival, the fear of living. Do this daily for a few minutes for 30 days. How do you feel, brother?

I feel very good. I would say I feel a renewed sense of confidence. Thank you.

Collect Sun Energy

Hinsurahamm: What does the Sun do? The Sun gives life for new beginnings. A seed planted in the ground and nourished by the earth and other elements cannot fully develop unless there is sunshine, so Sun energy is very critical in your awakening process. The Sun supports growth. If there were no Sun, none of the people, animals, or plants would be alive.

We want to tell people who are on the path of ascension to increase the frequency of their exposure to light. One way to do this is to collect Sun energy. Imagine you are breathing the beautiful, powerful energy rays of the Sun, and you draw them into your cellular structure. Your cells burst forth with the light of the Sun.

This can do two things: (1) It can expel all the energies embedded in your cells. (2) It can give you a powerful boost of energy. When you are tired, working with the Sun can boost your energy. You will feel less tired because the Sun will burn the fats causing you to feel drowsy and tired. Working with the energy of the Sun can rejuvenate you, regulate your metabolism, and kick-start a new energy inside you.

Many ancient cultures — Egyptian, Indian, Maya — worshiped the Sun. If you go to these places, you will see temples dedicated to the Sun god. They knew that without the Sun, they could not go forward. We, the dragon energy, support anchoring the Sun's rays into all humanity, especially during times of an eclipse. Solar eclipses are very powerful. Our energy is linked to the energy of the lion species, especially the white lion. White lions are a sacred animal, and many traditions have ceremonies of initiation with the white lions.

Just before Jesus was born, the most powerful rays of the Sun were anchored into the ground, preparing, cleansing, and beautifying the light. There was a lot of optimism, and there was a lot of fear, hatred, and anger. King Herod knew that a very special person would be born. There was much anger and anxiety among his people and in him.

We need to anchor a powerful spiritual light so that the land becomes pure for the master to be born there. You have read in other books that people have their own powerful rays connected directly to the Sun. Sun energy is connected directly to the silver cord between your pineal gland and the Creator. Working with the Sun dragon can help you to awaken this part of you.

This energy will become like a lamp that is always lit within you, a liberating lamp. Imagine a lamp always inside you continuously glowing. You will feel comforted. You will feel energy course through every part of your body, warming you, and you will embrace the beautiful love of your divine soul.

We have anchored our energy in a few places on the planet. This is why some places are powerful spiritual vortexes, and when people go there, they are uplifted and liberated. One such place is Boynton Canyon in Sedona, Arizona.

Native Americans have dances and ceremonies honoring the Sun, and they perform special ceremonies during eclipses. Other places we have anchored this powerful energy is under Mount Shasta, Stonehenge in England, certain places in Israel, the southern parts of India, and a place called Chennai in the temples of Madurai. We have also anchored energy in Brazil in the Amazon jungle and in certain Polynesian islands.

We anchored energies when the planet was created. There were master builders and other beings who placed important spiritual artifacts deep underground. These are cylinders that contain geometric patterns and writings, and they are buried deep inside Earth. Our energy supports their function in the fullest capacity. Some of them will be found in the future, but we encourage you to not touch them and to leave them in place. Many will not be found because they are buried deeply. They are key factors in maintaining Earth's stability.

Our work has become more critical because of what is happening to the planet because of people's chaotic thought processes and mining operations on Mother Earth's body. This has created a lot of instability. Extracting minerals and oil has caused her to lose balance. When she loses balance, the beings on her body also feel unsure and insecure, and they develop a sense of anxiousness or fear as if the other shoe is going to drop.

We are working hard to stabilize these factors, but on a personal level, we encourage you to call on us and ask us to anchor the energy of the Sun within you. Ask that all the codes and seeds within you be fully awakened. Let the seed of enlightenment be rooted deeply, and let it sprout and become a gigantic tree within you.

1.   The nucleus of your body is inside your bellybutton. Some cultures call this the sun chakra. Bring your energy to this place. Imagine a

white disk, a circle of light, around your navel. This circle of light is blazing beautifully. As you breathe, this circle starts spinning. It will go deep into your body. As you breathe, the chakra will spin faster and become bigger.

2. Slowly it will become bigger and overtake you, and you will be inside the circle of the Sun. Imagine the Sun is glowing within you. You will start feeling hot and sweaty, but when the Sun is active in you, you can throw away many unwanted energies from this lifetime and past lifetimes.

Many patterns and bad habits will be pushed off by the Sun. It is a warm, cleansing energy. When the Sun comes out, no lower frequency can remain there, for the Sun will burn everything. It is very, very strong.

Simply call on it, and activate this Sun disk within you. This is all that is needed. Anchor the Sun energy within you, and you will experience an uplifting energy instantly. Bring the Sun energy into your house to energize everything in there. Bring it to your work and to your relationships, any place you need it.

Access the Resurrection Flame

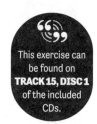

This exercise can be found on **TRACK 15, DISC 1** of the included CDs.

Dragon energy is connected to the resurrection flame — the rejuvenation, or the healing, flame, where we are one with the Family of God. Do you have any questions?

Could you elaborate on the resurrection or the healing flames? Where are they, and how can we access them?

These flames extend from your feet. Through them, you can resurrect your connection to the Earth spirit, for you must join with the Earth spirit for liberation. The Earth spirit supports you. It is a combined energy of all that is, and you need the support of the Earth spirit to move into ascension. This is accessed simply by focusing and calling on the resurrection flame to be activated.

1. Now close your eyes, and focus on your feet. The fingers of each hand are closed and touching the middle of each palm, except the index and middle fingers, which are extended and shaped like a V. Each thumb rests on the ring fingers [figure 14.2].

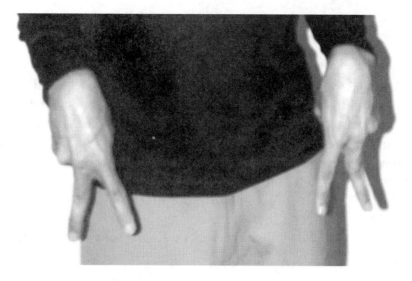

Figure 14.2. Mudra to activate the resurrection flame

2. Point both V's toward your feet. The right hand V points toward the right foot, and the left hand points to the left foot. Now breathe. Just keep breathing.

It seems like my breath is going out those two V fingers down to the feet.

Yes, and you will start feeling tingling energy or sensations on the toes.

I do.

3. Keep focusing. Close your eyes, and breathe. Imagine this beautiful white sunlight from your navel area. Breathe this light. Focus it. Inhale it, and send it out through your fingers to your feet. You will start feeling this immediately in your feet. You might even see flames in your hands. They're not hot. They are beautiful silver-white flames.

Yes. I can sense that.

4. Continue this, and slowly make the sound "gumm."

Gumm, gumm.

You are simultaneously making the sound and sending the energy from your navel into your hands and into your toes.

My feet are tingling away. Gumm, gumm.

You can chant this slowly in your own way.

[Chants "gumm" many times.]
You will feel energy in your fingers and toes too.

Yes, and my impression is that the purification is happening on the cellular level.

Yes, and it's also a release. When there is release, natural purification happens. Working with this every day, you can activate the energy of the resurrection flame and the healing flame. We combine these two. You are in a very powerful place.

5. You will see this flame move slowly into your forehead; there are energies of higher beings there, the Elohim. They are master builders. They can help you build your master plan. Call on them. The key to calling on them is activating the sun flame under your feet — also known as the resurrection flame, the healing flame.

Thank you. Somehow this makes great sense.

Balance Energies

Family of God: Now we invite the next dragon. This dragon holds feminine energy and form. She is the dragon of the Moon. Her name is Lamihh.

Lamihh: Hello, hello. We are holding the energy for the dragon called Lamihh, for we are a group energy here to support you by sowing seeds of the feminine within you — awakening the feminine within you. We are connected to the consciousness of the great mother, Isis. All cultures up to the present honored us. Many had ceremonies to honor us. Many cultures called us Mother Moon. There is great need for our energy to be embedded into Earth, for this planet is in a very precarious condition. It could turn either way. It could go to the right or to the left. This is a key concern at this time. We are working with other dragons to rectify this energetic imbalance.

One of the problems is the depopulation of fish in rivers and the seas. Because of fishing and pollution, the fish population is dying. When that happens, there will be much more turmoil on the planet. People will become more imbalanced and hardened. Their hearts will be stuck and not open to compassion or new ideas. We, the dragon collective, support the Moon and the moon dragon. We beam powerful energy into the waterways. We give messages through codes to fish to reproduce so that the waterways are kept clean and safe. This is very important.

Mother Moon rules and influences human beings. Emotions are supported by the Moon. Since you are a water being, the Moon has a very big influence on you. Work with the energy of Isis, for we are in complete harmony and union with the energy of the Moon.

Planets have their own moons. Since parts of you live on these planets, you are also being influenced by the moons of other planets, but this is not understood. You can understand this concept by dividing yourself into twelve parts. Only 8.25 percent of your existence and consciousness is on a planet. The rest is on other planets, so you are affected by the moons of other planets. You are having simultaneous experiences living in a physical body on other planets.

1. Our dragon moon energy is around your head. Imagine a band 3.5 to 4 inches wide around your head. This is a light-green color with a tinge of soft, shining white light. Breathe, and say, "limihh."

Limihh.

2. When you make this sound, this band will spin slowly around your head. It will come into you, and you will be inside this circle. It will go up all the way to the twelfth chakra and then descend. It envelops you, and it goes deep through your entire body and through your feet into the ground.

3. You are bathed in a gold and silver light with a tinge of white. Anchor this into the ground. This balances your emotional body and the water within you. So now we have the Sun energy and the Moon energy within you, both in a balanced way.

Initially when you do this, you might feel your head spinning, or you might feel spaced-out. When our energy comes into your auric field, it can balance many distorted energies in your aura. It will cleanse, purify, and release many unwanted belief systems and attachments — false attachments to the lower ego. When the false attachment leaves, you are liberated. You will say, "Why was I holding on to that? What good was it?" And you will be able to let go easily. False attachments will start falling away and be replaced with a sense of liberation and freedom.

Now, do you have any questions for us, brother?

No. I believe you explained it very clearly.

All right, then. At this time, we will take our leave.

Thank you.

Adjust to Change

Hinshio: Hello, brothers and sisters who read this. We welcome you to understanding the process of ascension using the energy of the dragon of the seasons. We are the energy of the Hinshio, supporting the changing of the seasons. These changes affect the human mind and human sight. Your body is attuned to the cycles of the Moon, planets, and changing times. Seasonal changes have a big effect on the growth and development of your physical organs, the energy in your body, and the activation of wisdom in your bloodstream.

The organs of your body undergo seasonal changes like trees. It is important to adjust to seasonal changes because your organs shift with the seasons. Some organs hibernate for a season, and their functions are filled by other organs. Some people work better in the early morning. This is because of the cycles of their organs.

The optimal time to meditate is around six o'clock in the evening. Your third eye is more open at that time. The pineal gland is more active between two and three o'clock in the morning. Your thymus is very receptive in the early morning as well.

* * *

Family of God: This completes the understanding of the dragons and how they can support you in moving forward on your ascension path.

Activate and Deactivate Ethereal Codes

The Family of God

Family of God: Hello, brother of light. We are the Family of God. It is always a warm feeling to reconnect with the family of humanity. So we say thank you for reconnecting and remembering once again.

This is a noble project. You are bringing forth important information. Today we share information about ascension key 15, code activation and deactivation.

The Yeshua Code and Crystalline Consciousness

Many codes need to be activated and deactivated for ascension. The crystalline code needs to be activated because of the shift that happened in 2012. The shift was about slowly bringing humanity into the crystalline grid rather than the magnetic grid. What does that mean? It means moving people from a lower level of energy centered on the base, second, and third chakras to a higher frequency. It does not mean that one chakra is above another. It means moving from base instinct to more critical thinking and then to a higher reality.

The effects of the magnetic grid are being lessened in the ground and in the human body. This means that people will be more open to change and will have clearer understanding. This is the next level to open inside you. It is called the crystalline consciousness from the crystalline grid.

You must open the code of the crystalline grid, which is represented by Master Jesus, or Yeshua. Simply asking that this code be activated signifies your acceptance of the crystalline light within you. It's a reconnection of the Christ child within you, representing the Second Coming of the Christ within each human being. This is a movement from magnetic to crystalline consciousness.

The Maitreya Code

Maitreya is the universal Christ consciousness on a much higher level. It encompasses many divergent realities. The Maitreya code is way above your head, and some representations of this code can be found in ancient Tibetan and Indian drawings. It is much higher than the 10th or 12th chakras. It goes up to the 144th chakra. This is about 4.5 miles above your head.

This code is not active in most people, and most people are not aware of it. If you are not aware of it, you cannot connect with it. If you did not know Mount Everest existed, you would never try to climb it. Once you know about something, you can make a goal and work toward reaching it. You would say, "I need to reconnect with this goal and draw energy from it."

To activate this code, do you simply ask for it?

Yes. When Earth was created long ago, there were master builders who came to the planet. Some came to the country you are in now, America, in a place you call New Mexico, and they set up grids using the power of sound and intention. This was done millions of years ago, so this planet was, for a time, in a much higher frequency.

At this time, we are moving higher and higher as well. This planet has a goal of attaining a higher frequency and moving into a higher dimension. This can take many years to accomplish. The master builder energy is collected through the Maitreya code in a human being, and these master builders laid grids in certain parts of the world, many in America and some in Peru. There are also some in Mongolia, some in Africa, and a few in China.

The Maitreya energy holds the energy of the first plane and other realities. But ascension happens in your physical body on the Earth plane, so it is good to connect with these grids. Once you know these grids, you can control the grid energy. Many of the grids are in America.

In the Southwest?

As well as many other places. There is one in Miami, one in Mount Shasta, and more in other places.

Corey Goode has been talking about the ancient builder race who inhabited this planet millions of years ago.[1] Are these the same people you are calling the master builders?

No. The master builders were commissioned by the Council of Creators regarding this planet. They were asked to lay grid lines, and then they left. There were master builders who came after that, but we are not talking about those builders. They are builders who came from other planetary realities. We are only talking about the master builders who came to set up the foundations here, along with dragons, before any human beings ever walked the planet.

Is it fair to say that these master builders were etheric beings and that they did not live as physical beings?

They were etheric beings, but some of them took physical form because that was needed. Lord Maitreya heads this division of the energy grid.

That grid is still in existence. Is that correct?

It is still in existence, and if more people come to know about this grid, it would become more active. Otherwise, it will remain dormant.

I would be grateful if you could tell me where, in the United States at least, these grids are located so that people can know and perhaps could take advantage of going there.

There are grids in Wyoming, Mount Shasta, the mountains of New Mexico, the mountains of Colorado, the mountains of Utah, Virginia, the upper highlands of New York, the Deep South near New Orleans, and Texas. Texas is a very special place. It has a lot of gruff energy, but there are temples, and there are pyramids. There are pristine mountains in Colorado, and when people go there, they feel very good.

1.   Learn more about Corey Goode at spherebeingalliance.com/blog/ancient-builder -race-recovering-humanitys-billion-year-legacy-part-1.html.

Other places include Lake Titicaca (Bolivia), Chile, and Mexico (the Sun Temple).

I believe it is called Teotihuacán.

Yes. There are grids in Bulgaria, and the Bucharest Mountains in Romania are very special. Also, there are grids in Tibet. Lord Maitreya is the head of this, so when you collect this energy, you can raise your energy. You do not have to visit these places. Simply intend to draw forth the energy and extend yourself to that place.

The Melchizedek Grid

The Melchizedek grid is not of Earth. It is etheric. It is in another reality. When you connect with the Melchizedek grid, you will join heaven and Earth through its energy. These three grids — the grid of Yeshua, the Maitreya grid, and the Melchizedek grid — will be able to free many incredible power shifts. These grids are important, and it is important to connect with them.

The Melchizedek energy is very strong in your thymus area, which is in the left side of your heart. Once you connect with these grids and activate the codes, you will feel an incredibly powerful energy within you. Once these three codes are activated, you will be in a shower of light.

The Lemurian Code

A code that needs to be deactivated is the Lemurian code. It will surprise people to know that this code needs to be deactivated because your origin is in Lemuria. Lemurians were very beautiful people, but they were one-sided. That means they were very feminine oriented, which is good and heart-centered, but they were not balanced. Balance means the mind energy must be balanced with the heart. They were very loving people, but that is only one side of the story. You must have both energies, not just one.

That is simply not appropriate for the current times.

Exactly. It is not appropriate to carry this now.

So to deactivate this code, we just ask for the code to be deactivated?

You ask with great intensity that this not have any energetic influence within you. It is done through intention. These codes were implanted from the Temples of Ascension in Lemuria. The priests of Lemuria were very advanced beings. They supported people, but there were also priests who felt superior to other people because they were a priestly class. They did not share all information with the people.

Similar things happen now. Secret energies kept some people feeling that they were better, so many people now feel they are superior because they hold secrets. We need to deactivate that. This is very deep inside.

The Atlantis Codes

There was dominance in Atlantis, a feeling that "I am special. I am superior." The latter part of Atlantis was more masculine. This influenced millions of people. This code is deactivated through intention, and by doing so, you heal the deepest part of yourself and balance your energies.

When you deactivate the codes of Atlantis, you also deactivate a guilt code: When Atlantis sank, many of the priestly class felt they were not able to help, and their understanding did not save the land.

Some priests left before the cataclysm but not everyone. And they carried incredible guilt that they were not able to save the temples, the people, or themselves. This happened among the priests of Atlantis. These codes are in your etheric bodies.

The Fear of God Code

A very important code to deactivate is the fear of God code. All people who have acted in the name of God believed they were doing what was right. Yet incredible injustices have been done in the name of God.

In other words, the fear of God was instilled by self-righteous people who believed they were acting for God?

In the name of God. God would punish them. Look at any religion or conquest. This energy is embedded in the navel of the physical body.

The Human Origin Code

There is another code that must be reactivated and strengthened — the human origin code. This code is important to connect with the energy of the original people who came to this planet in

Africa. These are human beings, not the ancient master builders. This is connecting with human origin on the Earth plane.

When people came here, they had full understanding and full memory, but over the course of time, this was lost. Because of Earth's density, even the ones who came with knowledge simply forgot because the density was very, very strong. This code is held in Mount Kilimanjaro, and in the human body, it is held between the knees.

Heal Physical Trauma from Former Lifetimes

The Family of God

Family of God: Blessed brother of light, we are the Family of God. It is truly an honor to communicate this way to bring forth understanding that can support people in these challenging times to come back into the light that they are. Thank you for holding this light.

Today we would like to talk about ascension key 16 — healing physical trauma of former lifetimes. Much has been said about the importance or, depending on the culture, the unimportance of the body and about how you can survive on energy alone to sustain your body. Much has also been said about people who are able to live long periods. The body is a finely tuned mechanism, a fine instrument, through which the soul expresses, creates, and re-creates experiences it intrinsically knows. It is important to understand that the body must also be prepared for ascension.

Your body contains pockets of energies stored in different places and in bodies in other realities. If your body has been abused or damaged in a past lifetime, your present body will contain the energies of those traumas and wounds. If your body had been traumatized by a fatal injury, your new body will contain energetic remnants of that injury. If your previous body was buried or cremated, its energy was not disbursed.

If there were serious bodily injuries in a past lifetime, you carry that damaged energy in your physical body. That must be healed, especially if the damage was through a traumatic death. The shock from those events will remain with you. It is in your energy field, and you will not be able to hold much light because your physical vessel contains that traumatized, dense energy. You have brought that energy into your present lifetime.

You can use divining rods to query whether you are carrying physical remnants of energy from the past five to seven lifetimes you had on Earth. Use your rods, and they will give you an answer.

Am I being influenced by energies from damage to my physical body in the past five lifetimes? Yes. I can see that the answer is yes.

This is understood very little. When you are born, you bring remnants of that energy into your body, so communicating with your body and releasing those imprints is critical to holding higher vibrational frequencies. This is one of the main reasons people are not able to maintain higher vibrational frequencies. It's because of the dense energy in their physical bodies. This will push out the higher frequencies, and the strongest energy will prevail. There is no space for the new frequency to come in and settle. For example, your muscles carry a certain frequency, so when you meditate, chant, or pray, you bring in good energy, but that energy just settles on the top layer. It cannot penetrate more deeply because of the dense energy from past lifetimes.

This is very critical work for ascension. As you work toward anchoring higher frequencies of light, you must anchor higher frequencies into your muscles, tissues, bones, bloodstream, hair, skin, nails, and teeth — every part — and ask that these parts transmute the traumatic energy you have brought from past lifetimes, up to at least five to seven lifetimes.

So we should not go further than five to seven lifetimes?

That will be enough unless your auric field is severely damaged.

For example, people who died during the bombings of Japan or people who were burned at the stake experienced dreadful traumas. Everyone watches as you burn and scream. In such a case, trauma could be very deep-seated, lasting 100 or more lifetimes.

So someone could use divining rods to determine whether that was the case?

Yes. You have to do this when there has been a horrific death in which the body was disintegrated, perhaps burned by fire, particularly if this happened while conscious. There could have been a wildfire, an explosion in an ammunition factory, or a bombing. When people die in these circumstances, all the spiritual wisdom they had gained in their evolution also disintegrates. Their souls have a hard time making up what was lost. The eternal soul does not die, but the soul has many realities and many dimensions. Their earthly, third-dimensional bodies are completely destroyed and, along with them, all the wisdom they had gained up to that point.

When you anchor light for ascension, you must anchor light into all your physical organs as well as the muscles, tissues, bones, blood, skin, hair, and nails. This is not understood by people working toward ascension. Yes, they are acquiring higher frequencies of light, but to fully anchor and go deep within, you must empty the vessel by clearing the tissues and organs.

May I ask a question now, please?

Yes, please.

I think I understand this, but I would like to clarify it. How is this key different from the second key, which is healing the trauma of soul fragmentation? You are speaking of damage to the physical vessel here whereas that is damage to the psychic vessel of the soul. Can you make that distinction?

Yes. Soul fragmentation happens when there is a traumatic death and the soul cannot take the pain or horror, so part of the soul leaves. Here, we are talking about the physical vessel. When you are born, although you have a new body, it contains remnants of the energy of the former physical body, so this is a matter of clearing up the damage that was done to former physical bodies. Usually doing this for five to seven lifetimes is sufficient, depending on the traumas involved, but sometimes it could be hundreds of lifetimes.

Work with Lord Melchizedek

I have heard or read somewhere that birthmarks are indications of old wounds from former lifetimes. Is that true?

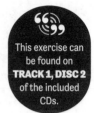

This exercise can be found on **TRACK 1, DISC 2** of the included CDs.

Birthmarks are important indicators of experiences in the psychosocial body from past lifetimes. It might be due to trauma or important rites of passage. In many cultures, religious ceremonies involved piercing the body. This was an appeasement to the gods, so a birthmark may not only be due to a traumatic experience. Where the body was pierced, the mark on the body can remain.

How can you work with this? The master of this universe is Lord Melchizedek. The universe is supported by many beings, but the master of this universe is Lord Melchizedek. You can call on this benevolent, loving being to channel his energies into your physical body. Ask that his energy go into all the Earth bodies you have had so far, at least up to seven lifetimes in Earth reality, and that his energy go into all your organs and tissues to be cleansed and transmuted.

You can also ask that all the energies in your bodily systems be transmuted — not just from physical injury, but also traumas of self-worth, trust, and faith. You can ask to be cleansed of manipulative behaviors, such as seeking validation, self-inflicted injury (physical or emotional) to gain sympathy, or excessively praising other people to feel loved or shown affection. All this must be purged, and Lord Melchizedek's energy can go into all these parts to transmute the energies of lack.

When you work with Lord Melchizedek's energy, releasing the energy of lack, you will awaken the energy of liberation. What is ascension? Ascension means liberation of yourself, the light, the truth, and the wisdom. It means liberation from the prisons you have built using your mind. Lord Melchizedek's energy is very gentle, but it has the power to go deep into the cellular structures and bring healing to everything we just mentioned. Too many people still believe, deep down, that they are not worthy or good enough for God, that they are not good enough for the abundance in life, and that they must suffer.

You speak great truth. If I understand this correctly, these issues or attitudes that you've outlined set up the physical circumstances that injure the physical body. Is that correct?

Yes. Because these energies are so strong in the tissues and organs, they create a reality on a day-to-day, minute-to-minute basis.

By clearing or diffusing the attitudes that you mentioned — unworthiness, lack of whatever — we can resolve the issues that are carried in the physical body.

Exactly, and when they are cleared, you will see a clearing in your mind as well. Your thinking will change because you have cleared the cause. When you clear the base, the top will change as well. You will feel release and liberation. You will be amazed when you realize that you were carrying all these dense energies you didn't realize you had. Everybody carries some aspects of these at some level. So many people seek acknowledgment from someone else. There is nothing wrong with acknowledgment, but just seeking it to satisfy a wounded part of you comes from a place of deficiency.

Working with Lord Melchizedek is like pouring liquid energy into your organs. You will see a huge difference. The beauty of it is being able to see the difference physically and mentally. Work with Lord Melchizedek's energy for 2 weeks, downloading it into your organs. It requires about 10 to 15 minutes a day.

1. Ask Lord Melchizedek to fill your organs, tissues, muscles, and bones — every part of you.

2. Ask Lord Melchizedek to anchor the energy of liberation into your navel: "I ask Lord Melchizedek to anchor the energy of liberation around my navel." This contains many of the emotional components through which you react and respond.

3. Ask that this area be completely cleansed and purified. See this energy as a vortex spinning in a beautiful metallic white around your navel. It will spin clockwise as viewed from the outside. Ask that this energy be anchored there permanently. You will feel a warmth in that part of your body. Close your eyes, and watch the white energy move around your navel. Just focus and breathe there. It is like a spinning white wreath. You can say, "I ask that this be anchored within me permanently."

I can feel it. I could feel him from the minute you brought him here, and I can definitely feel this.

Do you feel the warmth in your stomach now?

Yes, I do.

When you continue this, the warmth will spread through your body, and this warmth will give you love for yourself. This warmth has the capacity to transform anything, as heat transforms cold. Every time an uncomfortable situation happens, you can focus on your navel to fully activate this revolving circle. When it generates warmth, the experience will melt into that area. You will feel better very quickly. Why? The more you move into ascension, the more you get away from drama. You are able to resolve situations as they happen, not allowing them to linger.

Whatever comes up, clear it and move on. In this way, you will feel more freedom. Your soul always seeks freedom. You will stop procrastinating. You will move on. You will not stay in a space of disharmony. Your soul always seeks to move forward and not dwell on a problem. Take action to resolve things and move forward. When you move forward, you will always feel love for yourself. You will feel good in your body, and you will feel warmth.

These are two simple steps: (1) Anchor the energy of Melchizedek into the organs, tissues, bones, blood, skin, hair, teeth, and nails. They all contain energies and frequencies. (2) Anchor the energy of liberation into your navel area until you feel warmth. People who work on themselves spiritually will be able to feel this energy of warmth immediately in the first sitting. It will move. There could be tears. You will realize your self-worth. You will always catch yourself before you do something to please others. You will say, "No, I violate myself. I do not need to please other people." You will become self-aware. Slowly you will take back your power.

Your body exists in many realities and dimensions. There can be trauma in your body in other dimensions, and this might be why it is difficult for you to hold higher frequencies. You can ask to channel Lord Melchizedek's energy, his sacred spectrum of light. This light is known as "ihoo" light. It is known in the Jewish tradition as omega light, and it has sacred geometric patterns of miniature triangles. As you meditate, call for the ihoo or omega light, and see yourself covered in small sacred triangles, miniature white triangles. This will heal other-dimensional bodily injuries. The main body you must work with is the physical body you now have. Then move on to work with your other-dimensional bodies.

You also can heal issues of genetic lineage with ihoo light. The effect is limited, but you can say, "I heal the body I inherited through my family lineage." Ask that it be healed with Lord Melchizedek's light. You can make that provision when you use the ihoo light.

Heal the Four Elemental Bodies

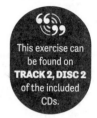

This exercise can be found on **TRACK 2, DISC 2** of the included CDs.

We will now talk about how your earthly body is connected to the Earth spirit. Your Earth body has four levels. One is the earth body, one is the wind body, one is the fire body, and the last is the water body. You can also include the etheric (or ether) body, if you like. You have these bodies in different realities. They are not on the physical plane. They are energetic signatures containing the same thought patterns and frequencies that you have in your physical body. When you heal your physical body, the other bodies are affected as well. The wind body is greatly affected, as is the fire body.

The beauty of this is that you can call on these four bodies to harmoniously integrate with your physical body because they contain four frequencies and qualities. You can call on these bodies to support you in solving everyday problems and issues.

1. Visualize that you are sitting in your physical Earth body, and on your right side is your water body. On your left side is your fire body. Behind you is the wind body, and in front of you is the ether body. Light is pouring into you. The light of the fire body is a soft orange-maroon color. The water body is the color of algae. The wind body is a very light purple. The ether body is soft turquoise.

2. Ask that these four bodies be fully harmonized with your physical body. Then you will be able to draw their strength whenever you need it. These elements are a part of you.

3. Bring Lord Melchizedek's light into the elemental bodies, and ask that they be completely healed, transmuted, and purified.

Once you become aware of the elemental bodies, imagine you are pulling them into you. You will feel more strength and power within you. You will become stronger. You will start acknowledging these elements within you, and they will support you because you have acknowledged them. This will open up the inside of you. You will become balanced on Earth in your physical body. You will become balanced with the elements. You will become balanced with the mind and the emotions. This understanding has not been brought forward before, but now you understand.

You know, it's simply amazing. It makes so much sense, and it is very elegant too. I like it so much.

You will see a dramatic shift in your search for ascension by working with the energy of Lord Melchizedek in your elemental bodies. You will be able to hold energy and accumulate it. Whatever you gain, you must keep and grow from that level and accumulate more. This is what ascension is. The more you anchor into yourself and hold, the more you will accumulate. If you work with Lord Melchizedek for the next 7 days, you will see a difference.

Lyme Disease

In the part of the world where I live, the northeastern United States, the land has become toxic to people because of a disease called Lyme disease. Ticks live in the forest, and people who go out there are bitten and pick up Lyme disease. It is difficult to detect, and it is very debilitating. I don't go out in the forest anymore. Part of the life cycle of ticks involves mice, and mice come into our houses. In the winter, mice carry the ticks. It has become very toxic. I'm wondering why this is happening and how we can heal ourselves if we get the disease. It is difficult to test for. For example, I had a client on Friday who has had this disease enter her cells, and she's traveling to Germany for two weeks to have a type of hyperthermia treatment in which her whole body is heated to 107 degrees to kill the spirochetes. This is something that is not done in this country. Can you speak about this?

This disease has spread far and wide, and the spirit of these ticks is very strong. They are telling human beings there is a cure for the disease. It has not been experimented with at this time, but when people are bitten by ticks and become aware of it right away, they can rub onions on that part of their bodies. They would be able to release a lot of the toxins transmitted by the ticks. The difficulty is that most people are not aware that they have been bitten or the tick has been in their hair. It burrows into their scalps, and sends poison into the body. Their cells are damaged.

You can work with the DNA in your signature cell, and this can change the frequency of your cells. This requires practice and knowledge, communicating with your signature cell and working with it.

For example, in your mind, you can inject the energy of raw onions into your signature cell [in your pineal gland], and visualize that this energy is going into all the cells of the body through your signature cell. But if the poison has already been there for a long time, this will not help. This only works in the initial stages, but it can definitely help. There will be a cure for this in about three and a half to four years.

As you say, many people are not aware that they have been bitten, and the antibiotic treatments are very spotty.

The antibiotics will not help much because they are only treating one thing. If a person is doing Chinese medicine or qigong or tai chi regularly, the energy in them will fight the spirochetes much more effectively. Working with a signature cell and the DNA can be effective.

I can tell you one more thing. Ask the people who come to you with this problem to deactivate the DNA of Lyme disease in their physical bodies. As you know, you are born with the imprints of all sicknesses in your physical body, and during the right circumstance, a disease can come forward. You carry those imprints, and you can ask to deactivate the imprints of diseases that you have contracted.

For example, a person may have had a full physical checkup but the next month have a heart attack. The person might ask, "Why didn't my doctor catch this?" The imprint was there for the heart attack when the person was born. It was part of his or her energy matrix, and the right circumstances (a word, an incident, an experience) brought the heart attack forward. You carry the imprints of all sicknesses. In the right circumstance, it can come forward. You can ask to deactivate the imprint of Lyme disease, but it must be done as soon as it happens, at least within the first few weeks.

We believe that there will be other herbal medicine treatments that can support releasing the poisons in the body, but they must also be done within three to seven days, before it gets into the bloodstream. In the future, there might be a vaccination. This is an avenue we wish for people to think about, consider, and experiment with.

Working with the signature cell can be effective. But there are other factors. First, you must believe in what you're doing because you are communicating with your body structure. If you do not believe in this and do it halfheartedly, it will not work. You must ask this question: Yes, Lyme disease is quite a strong disease, but how have the people in Brazil, living in the Amazon forest and other forests, been able to treat this?

Because they live in harmony with the land and with Earth, and we don't.

Also, they use herbal medicine.

Is this a synthetic disease, or has it always been around?

It has always been around. It is not a human-made disease. Lyme is a natural thing.

Balance the Nature Kingdoms in Your Body

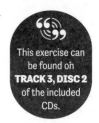

This exercise can be found on **TRACK 3, DISC 2** of the included CDs.

We believe you can gain support in your journey by working with the nature kingdoms. What do we mean by the nature kingdoms? Many say that the human body is a microcosm of the macrocosm. This means the entire macrocosm lives in your physical body, including the nature kingdoms. Nature, from our perspective, means mountains, rivers, forests, the earth, and stars. You must include them in balancing the energies within you. This is important because mountains, rivers, forests, stars, and the earth have a significant contribution to make to your lives here, and they formulate your path to complete the life tasks you have chosen for this lifetime.

These five energies are being sent into the ground, moment by moment, and from there, they are distributed to all human beings and other creatures, but human beings have the biggest effect on these energies. Once you balance these energies, you will also be balanced with the other elemental bodies.

The energies of everything on Earth, including animal spirits, exist within you. This does not mean you contain the energies of all animals but that the overall essence of the great thing we call animal spirits also exists within you.

1. Stand up, and keep your arms down at your sides so that your fingers touch your thighs [figure 16.1]. The forest spirit is on the left side of your body, and the mountains are on the right side. The spirit of the earth is beneath your base chakra between your thighs. Behind your body, you have the energy of the river. River energy is more important than the energy of the sea for human

beings because people are more closely associated with rivers than the sea. Above you is the energy of the stars.

2. As you stand, position your feet so that your right foot is in front of your left foot. Both palms are open, and your hands touch in the prayer position [figure 16.2]. Extend your arms in front of your body. Hold the prayer position, move them to the left side of your body [figure 16.3], and make the sound "saruu."

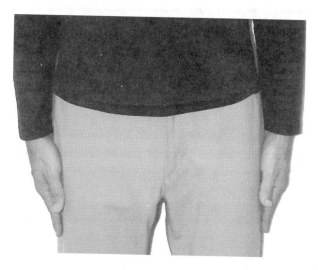

Figure 16.1

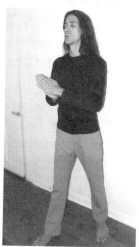

Figure 16.2

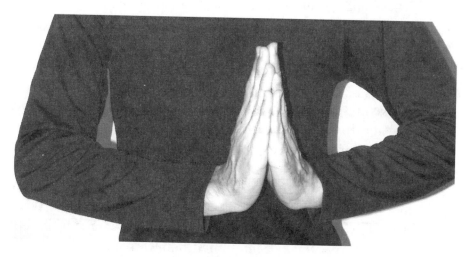

Figure 16.3

Figures 16.1–16.8. Mudras to balance the body with nature

Saruu, saruu, saruu. It is interesting. I can feel this energy going down the left side of my body.

Repeat this nine more times.

Saruu, saruu, saruu. Saruu, saruu, saruu. Saruu, saruu, saruu.

This will balance the energy of the trees within you. When the tree energy is balanced, you are in a much better emotional or mental frame of mind.

3. Now point your fingers toward the right side to balance the mountain energy [figure 16.4]. Chant "saruu" nine times.

[Chants "saruu" nine times.]

4. Now point below the base chakra between your thighs, and chant "saruu" nine times [figure 16.5]. This is to balance the earth energy within you.

[Chants "saruu" nine times.]

5. Now move your hands, in prayer position, behind you as best you can, and chant "saruu" nine times to balance the river energy [figure 16.6].

[Chants "saruu" nine times.]

You might feel some energy in the back of your body.

I do.

6. Now move your hands, in prayer position, above your head [figure 16.7], and make this sound to connect and balance the star energy in you. Chant "saruu" nine times.

You know, I can feel this. It's amazing. I'm getting visuals on this. Maybe you're suggesting it; I don't know. But I'm feeling these things.

Can you feel some energy movement?

Yes, absolutely.

Make these movements, and make this sound. It is simple. You will be able to balance these nature energies within you. They are part of the constitution of your body.

There is another sound. Keep your feet apart in the same position [right foot in front of the left], and bring your hands to prayer position in front of your heart [figure 16.8]. Close your eyes, and be in this space. Repeat three times: "aaummmeii, samwati, mehiiyuum, nantyozim, aren, aren, ringyo, ringyo, ringyo, manase, manase, manase."

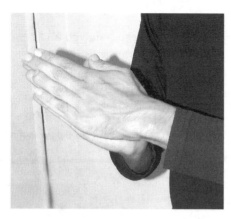

Figure 16.4

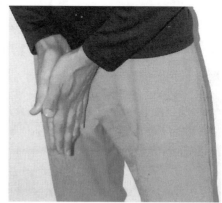

Figure 16.5

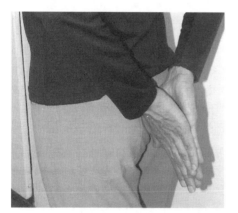

Figure 16.6

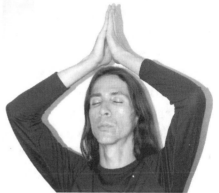

Figure 16.7

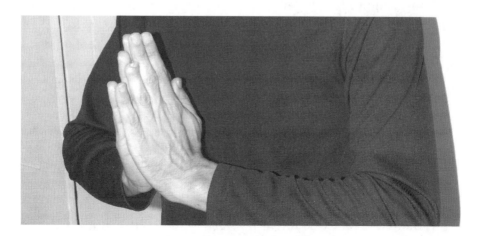

Figure 16.8

[Repeats the sounds three times.]

When you make these sounds, you will be able to balance all these elements simultaneously. Can you feel the energy building?

Yes, it feels very sacred to me.

Greet the Nature Spirits within You

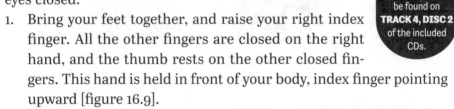

This exercise can be found on **TRACK 4, DISC 2** of the included CDs.

There is another exercise to do. Do this with your eyes closed.

1. Bring your feet together, and raise your right index finger. All the other fingers are closed on the right hand, and the thumb rests on the other closed fingers. This hand is held in front of your body, index finger pointing upward [figure 16.9].

2. All the fingers of the left hand are closed in a loose fist. The left hand rests comfortably on the left side of your body, arm down.

3. Bring your right index finger 1 inch in front of your forehead just above the third eye, not touching, so that your fist is level with your third eye [figure 16.10].

4. Make the sound "yaruu" three times. As you make this sound, do not sing it. This is a recitation. You speak it rather than sing it.

5. Bring your index finger in front of your right shoulder and say "yaruu" three times [figure 16.11].

6. Bring your index finger in front of your left shoulder, and say "yaruu" [figure 16.12].

7. Bring your index finger 1 inch in front of your navel, pointing upward, and say "yaruu" three times.

8. Point your index finger to the small toe of your right foot, and say "yaruu" three times [figure 16.13].

9. Point your index finger to the small toe of your left foot, and say "yaruu" three times [figure 16.14].

You have now covered yourself with the energy of these aspects of nature, and you are inside this energy. They are part of the protective energy field. You have anchored this energy throughout your body, and it will stay with you. You will feel it accumulate within you.

In human terms, this might not make much sense, but this is the language of nature, especially the trees, mountains, rivers, earth, and

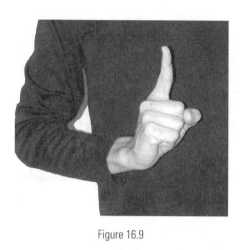

Figure 16.9

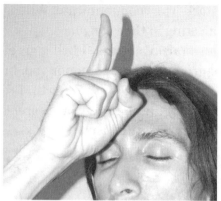

Figure 16.10

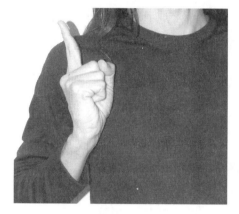

Figure 16.11

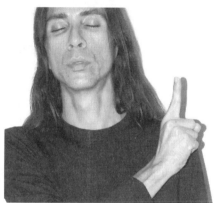

Figure 16.12

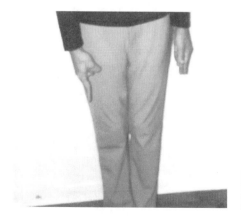

Figure 16.13

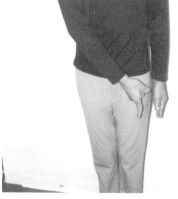

Figure 16.14

Figures 16.9–16.14. Mudras to greet nature spirits

stars. They communicate. When you use this sound, you are communicating in their language.

"Yaruu" means "I bring greetings to you. I deliver myself to the spirit of the trees. I honor you, brother mountain. I honor you, sister river, and you, Mother Earth, I remember you very well. I honor the spirit of the stars. I joyously greet all of you with my heart's love." This is very beautiful, isn't it?

It is very beautiful.

℘rogram
Sacred Geometry
of the ℱace

The Family of God and Jesus

Family of God: Blessed brother of love and light, we are the Family of God. What we bring forth through the support of you and Rae is important.

Ascension key 17 is about the eyes and the face of ascension. People have many characteristics imprinted on their faces. They have mouths, noses, cheeks, chins, and eyebrows. All these are centers of energy. When people see each other, what do they see first? They see the faces. And people make assumptions by looking at faces. If the face is beautiful, people are attracted, and if people find faces ugly, they are repelled. What does this have to do with ascension? Faces are constructed with geometric patterns. Some faces are round, some are oval, and some are elongated. Some people have long chins and long foreheads. Some have short foreheads, and some have lines on their foreheads. Some faces are chubby, and some are thin. All these characteristics are sacred geometric constructions.

Certain faces can attract more light. Other faces reflect karma. Your face draws people to you. Certain geometric patterns are powerful attractors. Which geometric pattern draws you? Is it an octahedron, a dodecahedron, or a tetrahedron? You are drawn to certain geometric patterns more than others. You will see that your eyes naturally go to certain geometric patterns. Certain facial characteristics can draw you into higher frequencies. Once you become aware of this, you can attract higher spiritual vibrations that exist in the ethers.

Your face contains the sign of a cross. There is a vertical line from your third eye to your mouth, and there is a horizontal line across your eyebrows. This cross interacts with the energies of nature, the stars, and the animal kingdom. To make this more complicated, you also have a pyramid shape at your nose. It forms a pyramid. You have a circle, and you have an octahedron. The circle is around your third eye, and the octahedron is circumscribed by the circle.

These geometric patterns are very sensitive to the frequencies around them. They move depending on your mental and emotional state. Let me give you an example. Suppose there are fifty people standing in line at an airport and a security person comes along and picks one or two passengers and asks to see their documents. They think, "Why me? Out of all of these people, what have I done?" The security person is able to see the movement in their faces. Because of stress or tension, these people hold those energies in their expressions, and the security person is able to see that something is wrong, so he or she singles them out.

You can raise your frequency to attract people. The next time you are in nature, open yourself to the energies of nature through these geometric patterns. You will feel more than what you see through your eyes. Feeling through your eyes happens through your geometric patterns. The geometric patterns in your face take on the geometry of nature.

Program Your Face to Attract Nature

When you are working toward ascension, it is important to connect with the earth and the elements of nature. They can support you. There are certain exercises that must be done outdoors because of the frequencies and energies available in the atmosphere. Your facial features will draw energies from nature. You can program them to draw higher frequencies.

You can connect with higher frequencies of the stars as well. You can call the energy of a galaxy or a nebula. Visualize a nebula. You are programming your face. It is like setting your antenna to pick up the patterns of the stars. Stars contain many geometric patterns. And this fine geometry is also contained in your face. This is why we recommend that you look at stars and spend some time in the evening under the night sky.

You communicate and interact with the stars through your sacred geometry. You can attune the geometry of your face with the geometrical patterns that appear in certain clusters of stars. Gaze at a star cluster that you are attracted to, and you will feel a download of energy from those stars go into your face.

Many ancient Indian and Tibetan masters gazed at the stars. Their eyes were frequently directed toward the sky. You do not need to name the star cluster that you want to attune to, but you can express your intention to attune to the energy of a star cluster with the geometry of your body. We recommend that you attune to the star Arcturus. You could connect with the Big Dipper and the Pleiades. You will eventually connect with stars that you have a special affinity to — Andromeda, the Pleiades, Orion, or Lyra.

Most people will feel the energy of the stars through their facial geometry within one to three sittings. Since these celestial bodies have a higher frequency, you will draw that forth. Human beings exist in all these places and all these star clusters. There is a part of you that exists there too. This is why you feel attracted to stars, and when you connect with them, you connect to a part of yourself that exists there. This is why people are attracted to stars. People like to look at stars. A part of you exists there.

You need to do this on a clear night. These are exercises that must be done every day, and once you get used to the energy, you can simply sit down in the evening in your room. Make the intention to attune your facial geometry to the geometry of a star. You will draw the energy of that star to you, so you do not need to go outside after you've developed a good connection.

Ascension energy is within you. It can be compared to watching television. You do not have to be at the television station to watch television. You just need an antenna or a cable. The cable or antenna for connecting with stars is in the geometry of your face.

See the Perfect in the Imperfect

The human body has so many more faculties than most of you know. It is a sacred tool designed to bring forth understanding and to help you grow. What about your eyes? It has been said that the eyes are the windows of the soul. When you fall in love with another person, you look into his or her eyes, and then you know. Eyes speak volumes. You can see love, compassion, and freedom, as well as the base energies of hatred, anger, and the instinct to kill when you look in the eyes. Communicate with your eyes daily to open them to see only truth and beauty — not only within you, but also in your surroundings, your brothers and sisters, and the kingdoms of nature.

Close all your fingers except the index and middle fingers. Your thumbs touch the ring fingers. Your index and middle fingers form V's. Bring your hands to your face. Hold your hands horizontally in front of your eyes so that the middle and index fingers of both hands touch each other [see figure 17.1]. Close your eyes. Now breathe. Breathe. You might feel some tension in your eyes.

I feel a lot of energy immediately. It's hard to describe, but it's like the vision of my eyes is being extended. My eyes are closed, but energetically they are extending.

You might see two or three balls of light. You might see planets and galaxies on that color spectrum. You are retraining and reprogramming your eyes. Yes, there is still ugliness in the world, and you will see ugliness, but you will also see beauty in the ugliness and the purpose of the ugliness, which exists separate from you. You will know that it is as it should be at this time. You are not affected by it. Whether it is good or bad, it is as it is. You will not judge.

You are reprogramming and reconstituting the energy of your eyes to exist without being left- or right-sided. Everything exists without judgment. This is where the masters live. A master might see a murder, or he might see a beautiful baby being born. A master blesses both events, knowing this is as it should be at that moment.

You see the world in detachment. You understand there is ugliness and cruelty, but you also understand that there is a higher purpose for what is happening. You only have compassion and acceptance for events, and you will do whatever you need to do in your power to support this, but you do not judge. It is as it is.

When a child is dying, a master will be with the child, knowing that

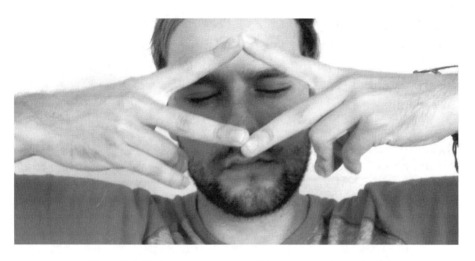

Figure 17.1. Mudra to program energy of the eyes to see beauty in all

the child is going to transition, and the master allows for the naturalness of the child to exist as it is in the moment. This is how masters live.
They exist completely accepting what is happening without judgment.
When you awaken and integrate ascension energy, you see through the
eyes of a master in an imperfect world, but you know you will exist as
perfect in this imperfect world. You know you are a lightbeing, shining
light into the imperfect world without judgment, and you love everything and everyone as a master. This is why eyes are very important.

See the World as a Master Does

The geometric patterns of your face are very important for ascension because the more you grow in light, the more compassion and
acceptance you have for the ugliness on Earth. This is called eyes
in ascension. When you start working with this, your perception
changes. Look at the masters. Embrace the beggar knowing that he
or she also contains the essence of God. This is a very high level of
mastery. This is what Mahatma Gandhi did. He stayed with the lowest of the low. He stayed with people who cleaned toilets. He ate
with "untouchables." He took an untouchable's name before he died
because he saw so much more than an untouchable person. This was
also Jesus's message. Jesus ate, slept, danced, sang, and drank wine
with the lowest of the low.

Truly advanced masters have this noble code in them because they have developed the eyes of God through their full awakening. They see beyond position. They see God in people, and they see the future potential that exists in everyone although it is not presently forthcoming.

Masters know the beloved soul of someone who is disabled or suffers from leprosy. They see people who have the potential to attain mastery. Masters see the highest potential in people rather than their circumstances. These are the qualities you see in masters — acceptance, tolerance, generosity, and the uplifting of other human beings at every possible turn.

People always ask how to raise their frequencies. It is very simple. Find five people every day, and make a commitment. "I will uplift these five people today." Upliftment could be by any means: making a telephone call, smiling, carrying a grocery bag, buying a cup of coffee for someone on the street, offering a seat to an elderly person standing on a train. You can always find ways to uplift people.

One of the main goals of masters who walked this planet was teaching how to uplift others. This was one of the themes of Jesus's teaching, uplifting other people. It must become a natural part of your life. By doing this, you add more and more light, and you uplift yourself. When you uplift another person through light, you increase your light. It is very beautiful.

It is very profound too.

Brother Jesus would like to say something.

Jesus: We, as spirit beings, are here every day listening to these mesmerizing conversations you and Rae have with the Family of God, so do not think you are alone. A thousand spirit beings listened to this conversation. This is the first time this information has been brought forth, and we are eager for it to be transmitted to and assimilated by humanity.

Each face has a subtle spectrum of colors imprinted on the forehead. This is why you are drawn to certain colors. When you observe a spectrum of colors, you prefer one color over others. You have a personal color spectrum, and you are attracted to certain colors.

We are not talking about the aura or the race of a person but rather the colors on the face. You can program your eyes to see these colors. People who can do this are called face readers. When they look at your face, they discern many characteristics about you. They understand colors and geometric patterns. They understand the mathematics of the face.

You can enhance your facial color to attract what you need. Think of expressions like "birds of a feather flock together" and "like attracts like."

There are eight colors in the human face: soft beige, pale white, subtle sky blue, pale leaf green, soft light brown, soft golden yellow, soft purple, and soft aquamarine. These colors can be enhanced. Breathe these colors into you. Be in front of a color, perhaps use a colored piece of paper or a flower. Visualize it, and breathe into it. This can enhance that color within you.

When you see a vegetable or a flower, the same colors in your face become very active. You are attracted to the flowers or vegetables of the same color. When you are at a party, you see men and women looking at each other, and some say, "I am hot for her" or "she is hot for me." The crisscrossing energy between these people happens because these colors are communicating. They are saying, "Let's join together and celebrate life."

Elevate Consciousness with Sound

The Family of God and Buddha

Family of God: We are the Family of God. When transformation happens, many are here to partake and hold the energies to support humanity. August is very special, as are September and October. A lot of energies are being downloaded, and they are bombarding people's minds. There can be times of cloudy thoughts. You will see how people react all over the world, from North Korea to Venezuela. The main energy being anchored at this time is unity consciousness. You can have unity first within you.

Having said that, we are now ready to discuss ascension key 18 — sound. Sound has the capacity to transform and elevate consciousness very quickly. Your thoughts are sound frequencies, and your soul hears those sounds. Your soul is very finely tuned, and it picks up subtle sound frequencies. Sometimes when you hear a sound, your body can go into shock. When that happens, the systems in your body that regulate the pumping of the heart, the functioning of the kidneys, and neural light frequencies going out of the brain are all affected.

Sound by its very nature is neutral, but the way you apply sound gives it form. Sound creates geometric patterns. Sounds made in pure love create geometric patterns shaped like snowflakes. Sounds uttered in anger or hatred create different patterns. The color becomes gray, and the shape is like a knot. Sounds uttered in pure love and compassion create patterns of circles and semicircles.

Since your body has many geometric shapes, imagine sounds creating geometric patterns that interact with the original geometric patterns in your body. Imagine that your body is a beautiful machine, and when you interject something that is not suitable for you, it will react. When this new geometric pattern is not in harmony, it will interact with the original sacred geometric patterns and greatly affect them. They cannot perform their functions freely or do what they were intended to do. This is why it is important to think and speak wisely. Wise people know that sound creates frequencies.

When you go to a church, temple, or concert hall, often you feel uplifted by the sounds because the music is creating beautiful geometric patterns that are in harmony with the original geometric patterns inside you. Ancient sounds and tones are very beneficial.

The parts of your body resonate with different sound frequencies. For example, sounds that benefit your brain are very different from sounds for your toes. There are sounds that create harmony, support your healing, and cleanse your bloodstream. This has been demonstrated by Dr. Masaru Emoto [see his book *The Hidden Messages in Water*]. When you communicate with water with love and thankfulness, the water molecules change. In the same way, when you make sounds with harmony and compassion, you feel lifted.

Sounds for the Heart: the Sarangi

The sound for the heart is from an instrument called the sarangi. This is a stringed instrument played with a bow, like a violin, but it is shaped differently. It is an ancient instrument used to perform ragas. It is still used frequently. Often it is played at night before people go to sleep.

The sarangi can soothe and heal a broken heart. If you ask whether it can support every human being, we would say yes. It will support you depending on your cultural beliefs and the attitudes you carry about music. (These can cause variations.)

Sounds for the Solar Plexus: the Morin Khur

The solar plexus is the nucleus of your body, and the instrument to support this is the morin khur. This instrument can bring an awareness of the positive in which you are able to balance yourself and come into a place of being positive in everything. It balances every area of your life — first within you and then with your family, work, children, money, spare time, relationships with friends and colleagues, connection to the Earth spirit, and connection with Father Sky. You will gain a clear perspective and start seeing things differently. You could realize, "This is the time I need to spend with my spouse," "this is the time that I need to spend with my children," or "this is the time I need to spend by myself for my personal growth; this is my time." You might realize, "I need to spend time with my friends."

You will gain a clear perspective, and your priorities will shift in a very beautiful way. You will not be as rigid. You will try to balance things. This is the principle of feng shui, in which you balance every area of your life. The sounds of this instrument can slowly bring this awareness and perspective to your life.

Sounds for the Spinal Column: the Lute

Your spinal column is an interdimensional tube that contains larger aspects of you — the larger truth and your essence. It contains past, present, and potential energies. When you work with these energies, the past can change your present, and the present can change your future. There are also chemicals in your spinal column and karmic energy in the form of fluids. When the spinal column is blocked, that means you are asleep, and it is difficult to awaken your kundalini. Energy cannot move through the density of a blocked spinal column.

The spinal column acts on your head as the stem of a lotus flower. The stem must be thick and strong for the flower to be strong. If the stem is weak, the flower is weak too. The instrument to benefit the backbone and the spinal column is an ancient instrument from the Middle East called the lute.

Sounds for the Eyes: the Levai

The instrument that is beneficial to the eyes is called the levai. This instrument can soothe and relax your eyes. When your eyes are soothed and relaxed, so is your body. This also opens inherent qualities associated with your psychic abilities — clairaudience and clairvoyance.

Under your eyes, you have portals to the asteroid Ceres. These portals are at the lower edges of your eye sockets, where your eyes meet the skull. Close your eyes, and bring your right hand's index and middle fingers together. Place your

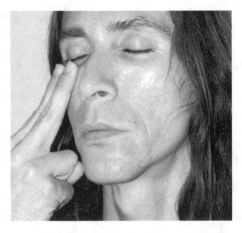

Figure 18.1. Mudra to relax your eyes

fingertips at the bottom of your right eye socket. Hold your fingers there, and breathe, moving your fingers gently [figure 18.1]. You will see light in your peripheral vision. You will feel movement there. You might also feel a slight headache or as if you are a little spaced-out. You might feel as if something is moving in your third eye. Very gently, move your fingers. Repeat this mudra with your left hand and eye.

Yes, I'm starting to feel that now.

Can you feel energy there now?

Yes, in the third eye.

This is the portal to the asteroid Ceres. When your eyes are relaxed, new realities open. You will be able to experience, see, and perceive a new reality. Otherwise, when a new reality appears, you cannot see it. You can only see the surface, and at times, you might discard what you see as a trick of your mind and ignore it.

Very few people are fully aware of their surroundings. When you climb stairs, how many steps do you take? You do not know because you are not aware. You live as an automaton. When this area of your eyes opens, you become aware of your surroundings. You know that there are spirits everywhere, and you become aware of them. Your response is very different.

You will honor your surroundings. You will not walk past a flower. Instead, you might stand there for a few seconds and appreciate its beauty. When you are unaware, you will not see it and simply walk by.

When you relax your eyes, you will notice the flower from your inner awareness. Sound can support your eyes to heal, relax, and see.

Sounds for the Stomach: the Gong

The gong is a very powerful instrument. It creates incredibly strong vibrations in your body, both front and back. It is especially good for your stomach, including the lining of your stomach. It is also good for your lungs, diaphragm, and kidneys.

Your stomach is an important area for your emotional body. It is the strongest part of your emotional body, and its nucleus is in your navel. When your stomach is strong, you will feel a sense of security and confidence. You will not be pulled down by everyday worries. You will see your life from a higher perspective.

Of course, there will still be challenges, but you will not be influenced by little challenges. You will say, "I will take care of this and move on."

When most people face a problem, they stay in the space of the problem. Suppose a mother gets angry and scolds her child. The child might say, "I'm sorry. I will not do that again." But the mother obsesses about what the child did for hours, and she goes on talking about it as if time has not passed. The incident is over, and the energy of it has left, but the mother remains in the same space. She is arresting her growth, and this is dangerous. This is not only an obsession; it is a karmic pattern she has brought with her. It is a self-defeating mechanism. She is holding on, and through this, she thinks she gains power.

There is an ancient story about two monks who had to cross a small river. They saw a woman sitting nearby who could not swim. She was afraid to cross the river.

The elder monk said, "Sit on my shoulders, and I will carry you." He dropped her off on the other side, and the monks continued walking.

After some time, the young monk said, "How could you touch a woman and carry her? You are supposed to be a monk, not a regular person."

The elder monk said, "I dropped her off at the riverside, but you are still carrying her with you."

People are like that, and because of this behavior, they don't grow. They block their energetic movement. Almost everyone has this tendency to some degree. People get stuck in a thought pattern and stay there, feeding the thought. Thoughts are powerful. They take on a life of their own and create a strong reality and an energetic imprint. People create their demons this way. This might be a reason people have stomach cancer. This condition is like a demon eating them alive because they have refused to let things go. They hang on to old griev-ances and get stuck in that energy. It is important to move on.

Listening to the sound of a gong and bringing this energy to your stomach can be very supportive in releasing thought patterns. Ascen-sion truly means releasing all that does not support you and coming back to yourself. And that is love.

Sounds for the Knees and Thighs: the Angklung

There is a beautiful instrument called the angklung. This instru-ment works directly with the spirits of your physical body, for your body contains many spirits. Many are in your bones.

Your knees are very important because they support your weight. They support your ability to move, and they give you the courage to be in the world and face its challenges and to heal and balance your karmic energies. When your knees are strong, you are fearless, and you walk with courage in your heart.

This energy is associated with the celestial horse. Many cultures depict this in paintings as a white horse. In India and Bali, you see a master riding a white horse, representing new beginnings, explora-tion, adventure, and fearlessness, raring to seek new pastures. In the Hindu scripture called the Mahabharata, Krishna speaks to Arguna. They stand on six horses that represent the chakra energies. These energies are connected to your knees and thighs.

When you are courageous, you are ready to explore new things. In your case, Robert, when you were younger, you had more courage than you do now. You journeyed to Africa. This courage enabled you to do more things.

Sounds for the Brain: the Rainstick

Your brain is a complicated organ containing many chambers and many parts. People talk about the higher brain, the God brain, the left brain, and the right brain, but there is more than that. There are many chambers inside the brain. There are energies of higher-dimensional realities, especially the energy of Andromeda. Your brain is not just for thinking and calculating. You can organize your brain to produce something magnificent. Thought is important, but if you organize your thoughts using sacred geometric patterns, you will be able to create something magnificent.

Imagine a golden ankh inside your brain. You can visualize this when you meditate, and you will see a shift in your thought patterns. This will help you find answers when you are searching for a solution. Your brain is connected to the celestial golden eagle. This represents your ability to soar into new heights and create freedom.

Your brain can be supported by an instrument called the rainstick. It is from South America. Its sound can reset the thought imprints of your brain, activate the DNA at the center of your brain, and act as a massage for a shrinking brain, which happens through distrust and faulty thinking. You can listen to this sound after you finish a bath. Nighttime is recommended, before you fall asleep.

Your brain will be completely attuned to use its different chambers — the left, the right, the third brain, the fourth brain, and so on — because your brain also exists in other dimensional realities. Your brain exists in your galactic body, solar body, universal body, and multiuniversal body.

Sounds for the Ears: the Xun

The sound to benefit your ear is from an instrument called the xun, which comes from China. Your ear is connected to your tongue, to the DNA in your mouth, your emotional body, and your body's meridian points. When these are activated, you are able to perceive the sounds of nature. These sounds are very therapeutic and healing. When you hear the sound of a cricket at night, you can perceive a higher reality or have a transcendent experience that spills into its chirp. This affects your DNA.

A cicada makes the sound "ki-ki-ki-ki" repeatedly. When you meditate on this sound, it can take you to the darkest corners of your mind, and from there, you can say, "I am ready to transcend now." But this can be frightening because it can bring out the dark parts. There are chakras behind your ears. Releasing the blocked energies in your meridians is a prerequisite to holding higher frequencies in your body.

Sounds for the Hips: the Didgeridoo

Regular bowel movements originating from the area of your hips are very important. This means that you are not storing energy. If you do not have proper bowel movements, you can create poisonous gas, affecting other parts of your body. The sound to heal this is made from the didgeridoo, an instrument from the Aboriginal people of Australia. These sounds can help your elimination process.

There are two DNA strands in your hips, and when they are activated, you have the natural ability to navigate through the world easily and effortlessly. This DNA is shaped like two golden screws. When you activate this DNA, you are naturally grounded in the world, and material manifestation can happen quickly. You are a grounded person, and you take grounded action.

When you do this, you might experience pain in your thighs. Pain happens when there is resistance in receiving. There may be pain because the DNA for this exercise has not been activated, and energy has never moved through these areas. Close your eyes, brother, and imagine two golden lights on your thighs and breathe in. See this golden light go into your thighs deeper, deeper, and deeper. Your breathing goes deep. You might feel some discomfort, but you will also feel a sense of security, groundedness, and certainty.

I am feeling the latter.

So this instrument is very good. It is best used in midafternoon, between 12:00PM and 3:00PM. There are no set rules; this is only a suggestion. You can follow your heart in doing this.

Sounds for the Face: the Harp

The harp has been called the instrument of the gods. There have been many cases in which people with serious heart ailments were healed listening to the sounds of a harp.[1] A broken heart can be comforted with harp music.

There are many chakras in your face, and there are three portals there: in your nose, under your eyes, and on your chin, where you

---

1. For an example of the healing powers of the harp, see boston.cbslocal.com
    /2016/12/22/harpist-touches-hundreds-of-lives-at-brigham-womens-hospital/ or
    https://www.ncbi.nlm.nih.gov/pmc/articles/PMC3863466/.

have a portal to the Pleiades. While listening to harp music, focus on your face, and be still for 15 minutes. This can help stabilize and recalibrate the energy of your face.

How many emotions can be displayed on a human face? There is a temple in Kyoto, Japan, with hundreds of standing Buddha statues. Each statue's face has a different emotional imprint. Buddha taught that you can choose to display the emotions you want on your face. If you were to enter a train with a frown, how many people would speak to you? On the other hand, a smile is an invitation for communication.

Body language will indicate whether someone is being truthful. Your body reacts to the emotions you display on your face. Once you master this, you will draw similar experiences into your life through the law of attraction. This is what Jesus did, and this is what the Dalai Lama does. You can deliberately choose the expressions you want to exhibit. When Jesus did this, people flocked to him, as they do to the Dalai Lama. This is a level of mastery. The harp can balance and heal the energies in your face and open the chakras there.

Sounds for the Arms, Elbows, and Hands: the Danuso

The sound frequency of this instrument can improve your eye-hand coordination, and it can improve your abilities to think, take action, and take a break. The healing chakras in your palms and under your fingernails can open with the sound frequency of this instrument.

Your elbows contain many secrets. Play this instrument while focusing on your hands, and your hands will become instruments of magic. The angel Cassien can help you with this. In twenty-five or thirty years, magic will become a natural expression for many people. This is the natural order of things, and it will start with the hands.

Sounds for the Legs: the African Drum or the Japanese Taiko Drum

The sounds these drums make resonate with Earth's frequencies and the chakras on the soles of your feet. Balancing the energies of your legs can help you feel in command of your life. Your perspective on life will change. You will take responsibility for your life without a sense of failure. You will not see your life as a win-lose game. You will look at life as an experience of creation.

You will like some of what you create, and you will enhance that. You will not like other things, and you will let them go. You will start looking at things differently and value things differently. You will value yourself more: "This is how I want to experience my life right now. This is my inner truth now." You will not judge what you do as a failure or a success. Everything will be an authentic experience.

Create Your Personal Sound Frequency

We have now covered all the instruments. For ascension, it is not necessary to work with all of them. Work with the instruments corresponding to the part of the body where you feel congested energy. Most people have congestion in some areas. Some people have more in their stomachs, legs, shins, and minds. Work where you feel you need healing.

The sounds you hear affect you. The sounds you hear when waking, when driving, when in nature, as a car passes, in an office, when brewing coffee, while riding in a train, or when a big truck passes all affect you.

You can isolate yourself, blocking all communication with your ears so that you do not pick up sound frequencies or resonances that are not in harmony with your body. However, we recommend that you make your own sounds every morning when you wake up. It can be any sound. Make that sound, and be with it for 5 to 10 minutes. Be in that energetic space. This is best done in the early morning before you drink coffee. When you wake, let the sound come from within you. This will create your foundation for that day.

When you are protected by your sound frequency, in a few days you will notice many sounds resonating within you, and the other sounds that you have been used to hearing — from your radio, iPad, or phone — will not resonate. You might lose interest in the pop songs on your car radio because they are not in harmony with your vibrational frequency. You will switch to a different type of music. You will switch to different sounds. You might still listen to some types of pop music, but it will be much more in harmony with your personal frequency.

So you will naturally choose things that are in harmony with your frequency?

Life is a choice, is it not? When you go higher and higher, you choose everything, and you are only going to choose what supports your frequency. You will not listen to music that brings your vibration down. You will say, "At one time, I enjoyed that, but it does not support me now."

You will see your eating habits change as well. Many foods you once ate will not appeal to you anymore. They are not necessarily bad for you, but you won't want them. You will start eating more natural foods, and you will eat less. The heavy, dense foods will lose their appeal. You might eat some but not regularly. Everything will shift and change. Your reading habits and your television-watching habits — everything — will shift. Sound is the key. You will move in tune with nature's sounds.

The key is making your own sound in the morning. Try it out tomorrow when you wake up. Don't feel shy. Let any sound come out through your voice. That is how you make your own sound frequency. It's pretty intuitive. Just express what comes out.

This will build energy around you. You will be in a bubble of this energy, and the other sounds you hear — when you go to the supermarket, talk with friends, interact with the plumber, or visit with your neighbor — will not have much of an effect on you. This will take some time to internalize, but you will notice the outside noise filter out. You are in your own sound frequency. Of course, you might still hear someone babbling on, but it will not have the same emotional impact on you.

I am fortunate that I have my own house, and it is set apart from other houses. But for someone who lives with other people or who lives in an apartment building where other people are close by, how would they go about doing that?

They need to create their own sound frequencies even if they are living with others, and then others will not affect them. They will be in their own energy field. They can do this quietly, even by humming. Do this for a minimum of 10 minutes. Make any sound that comes out from your deep self in the morning. You will see that each day different sounds will come out. One day you will pick one sound and say, "This sound really makes me feel good. It gives me passion and love." Then you will have found your individual tonal frequency.

So it's a trial-and-error process to some extent?

In one week, you will be able to find your tones. This tone will protect you. It will protect your house or your apartment. It will protect your energy field. It creates a bubble around you that no other energy can penetrate. Your energies will block that. You are creating protection. Has it not been said, "You are God"? Indeed.

Yes, it has been said, and I find that very beautiful.

Each culture has certain sound frequencies. Look into that. For example, the choral music of ancient Russia is very beautiful, or listen to music from Chile. You have lived in those places. Connect the dots, and you will find beauty everywhere. It can balance you.

When you use sound from other cultures, there is a reason. You will be calling your soul fragments from another lifetime. You might be able to say, "I don't know why, but I feel very much like listening to old European music," for example. This means at that moment, your soul is connecting to the soul fragments of that lifetime. You can choose something else later. Because you had lifetimes in other places, you will feel resonance with the songs that you listened to in those past lives.

You can also hear the sounds of Lemuria and Atlantis. There is channeled music from those places, and you can feel the resonance. There are sounds of a pyramid, a cloud, a rainbow, or a dragon. You should keep a journal. Write down which sound takes you far, which sound makes you feel integrated. When you get used to the sounds of your voice and your soul frequency, they can be used to create magic.

Blessings. We are the Family of God. Do you have any questions, brother?

I asked my questions as we covered this material. What you have said is amazing. I think it is profound. I have nothing but admiration. Thank you.

Self-Acceptance

Buddha: Hello, my brothers and sisters from all around the world. I am Master Buddha. What was given about sound is profound. Even my name, Buddha, is a sound frequency. My given name was Siddhartha. Jesus's name was not Jesus. That is an adopted name that supports the energy frequency he created, and he became that frequency. I suggest that you choose a name with an appropriate sound frequency to support who you have become in your spiritual evolution.

Certain flowers respond to sound more than others. Brother Robert and brother Rae, we would like you to work with their petals. One flower you could use is the soft-yellow rose. You will feel a sense of deep peace and deep love. Perhaps someone could help you. Lie down, and someone could place a petal above your third eye, another on your navel, and one on your shin, or if it won't stay there, put it beneath your feet. Just breathe with these petals, and focus on them. Slowly you will feel the scent of the petals within you. You will feel the very essence of the rose. The essence of this flower is beauty, love, and self-acceptance.

Lack of self-acceptance is one of the predominant causes of suffering. You want to be like somebody else. You do not accept yourself because you do not love yourself. If you are going to love another person to the fullest, you must accept who you are. Self-acceptance is a very important key in the ascension process. Flowers can support you with this.

We have said many times that there are energies of higher frequencies in your hands and in your chakras. There are healing energies in your hands. The energy of Mother Mary is there, and the energy of the creative force is in your hands. You also have something else in your hands. It is the energy of the three gods of India: creation, preservation, and destruction — Brahma, Vishnu, and Shiva. Open your hands, brother, and say, "I ask to experience the energy of the three entities Brahma, Vishnu, and Shiva in my hands now."

I ask to experience the energies of Brahma, Vishnu, and Shiva in my hands now. It's pretty amazing.

Can you feel the energy in your hands, my brother?

Oh, yes, immediately. It's hard to describe, but it felt like, not powers, but projections out of my hands that went upward at least a foot. There were energetic constructs. As I said, it is hard to describe.

Now this is important because when you activate this energy in your hands, this is the time you can take action — beautiful action — to manipulate reality. You will also know how to preserve it and when to let it go.

In the past few days, Bill Gates, the richest man on the planet, gave away $4.6 billion in his company's stock. He created this money, he preserved it, he encouraged it to grow, and then he let it go — Brahma,

Vishnu, and Shiva. At that level, life becomes fun. You say, "I am creating. Maybe I'll keep it and hold it for some time, and through that, I will grow. But I will also let it go." Life becomes fun.

Creating, keeping, and letting go — the three entities, the three energies — this is the cycle of life: creation, birth; preservation, living; destruction, death. It is a continuous cycle. When you are in this space, brother, you enjoy everything, but you know this is not you. Be in the world but not of it.

ᴀ𝒜ccess
𝒥𝒻eart 𝒲isdom

The Family of God and Master Mahareya

Family of God: Hello, brothers. We are the Family of God. We are sharing interesting experiences today.

Earth recently experienced an important eclipse — August 21, 2017. We wish to remind you that although the eclipse happened on a certain day, the journey of the eclipse took a long time to come to this place. It came from very far away, and its astrological appearance was perfectly timed.

We thank the citizens of Earth for joyfully embracing this in celebration, for we see this, and we note the festivities all around the world, including in Pakistan and other countries. This was a special astronomical event. Although people did not know it, they still felt something substantial had occurred. The excitement built energy for positive change.

Could you briefly explain the significance of this eclipse? I have ideas, but I'd really like to hear it from you.

This is a time you can make positive changes. Intentions expressed aloud are picked up by the Sun. They will be recharged with Atman particles of God and downloaded into the cells of human beings. This is called a manifestation.

A few weeks ago, a new energy called the aurora was downloaded. This represents the consciousness of prosperity and abundance, and it was delivered into the ground and activated in the codes of Mother Earth's body. The eclipse marked a time when people could make positive changes in their lives. By meditating on an intention, people bring healing to themselves and collectively to the planet. That is why this was such a significant event. It was widely visible across North America because North America is in the middle of a Pandora's box, and when changes happen there, they affect every part of the world. There could be some dramatic changes, even in the country's political situations.

Yes, and the internet is ripe with all kinds of things going on in this country.

Will the president leave, or will the president stay? Will there be more problems like what happened in Charlottesville, Virginia [white supremacists vs. progressives]? This is a time when positive changes can be made. Even though the eclipse is over, the energy remains. You will be able to remain in a meditative state for a time. People will still be able to make quantum changes relating to consciousness.

Okay, dear brother. Thank you. Now we come to ascension key 19 — the wisdom of the heart. We invite other masters to speak about this.

The Wisdom of the Heart

Master Mahareya: Hello, blessed brother. This is Mahareya. We embrace you in divine love. We embrace you in divine creativity. We embrace you in divine grace and compassion.

The human heart is a very delicate organ, and it has extraordinary wisdom. It has been wisely said that home is where the heart is. It not only keeps a human being alive but also directs the flow of love through the human body and into the ground and then out to the cosmos. The heart is not just a pumping machine. Through the heart, you can experience a meeting with the Divine. You might have heard people say, "Stay in your heart but with wisdom."

The heart has twenty-four chambers, and each chamber holds a certain frequency. Each is like a doorway, and the twenty-fourth chamber is your inner sanctum. In a large temple complex, a statue of the divinity or the inner sanctum is not at the entrance. It is almost always placed at the back of the complex. The twenty-fourth chamber is where your divinity resides. This is the place of your I Am presence. It is where you go during sleep to rejuvenate and heal.

We encourage you to go to this chamber daily, for this is your sanctuary. It is your holy and sacred place. Imagine a door opening into your heart. You enter and walk down some stairs. Each step takes you further and further in, and finally you come to the twenty-fourth chamber. A door opens, and you are in a beautiful golden space. This space was created for your I Am presence. You are greeted, comforted, nurtured, and supported.

The twenty-fourth chamber has sacred passages. Through these passages, you are able to access the consciousness of higher realities. This chamber is where you can visit and rewrite your akashic record. You also can request an audience with your guides, the Karmic Council, and the Council of Creation — all who support the movement toward planetary ascension. We entreat you to visit this chamber.

Your heart is not just in the front of your body. It is in the back as well. The energy of your heart is all around you, and it becomes enhanced when you feel positive. Your heart is not just about love but also wisdom. When there is love, there is wisdom. This wisdom will lift humanity.

Through wisdom, you will be able to move higher and higher. Through your heart, you will understand other realities and the oneness of all creation. Through your heart, you are able to perceive love, for your heart has love for you and for others.

Your heart also contains DNA. The Pleiadians gave their DNA to humanity. It is shaped like a pyramid, and it is situated below your sternum on the right side of your heart. There are secret chambers where you can access the realities of the mystical world, the magical world, and the world of make-believe. In these places, you have the potential to liberate yourself. Simply ask your heart every day, "My heart, tell me how much you are open today. Are you open fully? If not, why? What is troubling my heart?"

Make friends with your heart, communicate with your heart, and massage your heart. Because of stresses and tensions, your heart becomes condensed and shrinks. Visualize that you are taking your heart out and massaging it so that it returns to its original shape. See it bathed in a beautiful golden-white light.

Ask for all the spiritual supporting energies available to you — your guides, angels, ancestors, and others who support you — to surround you in a beautiful room. This is a place where you can request past soul imprints be rewritten and the cause of the suffering in your current lifetime be rearranged so that you do not have to go through a period of intense pain.

Interestingly, every country has a heart. North America's heart is wounded right now. When the heart is wounded, there is suffering, and when there is suffering, there is violence. Suffering and violence are synonymous. If you want to end the violence within you or your country, end the suffering. Suffering is caused by wrongful thoughts, thoughts that are not aligned with your soul. If you do not control your thoughts, your mind will take away your peace, and you will suffer. You suffer when you hold on to thoughts.

Ask What Makes the Heart Glow

Your heart is the place you can ask to reset your energy and prioritize the focus of your life. Brother Robert, ask your heart, "What makes my heart glow?" The answer is often not what you have in your mind. People say that their hearts glow when there is love or when they have abundance or good health. But many times, the answer will be unexpected. These things are important, but something else is more important for your heart. What is your answer, brother?

Well, I'm not 100 percent sure of this, but the impression I have is being of service.

Exactly. This is what we were going to say. Now you wonder, "How can I be a light unto that? How can I be a servant to humanity?" Do you see the difference, brother, how your heart glows in service?

You will see an expansion of your heart's energy in service. You will feel less violence within you through conflicting thought processes.

Imagine that there is a supercomputer inside your heart. It has two buttons. One is the delete button and the other is the save button. When you see an image of suffering, push "delete." When you see an image of service, push "save." This makes an impression in your heart that will stay there. This will become your truth, and since the image is saved there, it will be distributed throughout your body by the circulation of your blood. You can do this right now, and you will feel expansion. Are you ready to do this experiment right now, brother?

Yes.

Let's say you want to rectify or change something about yourself. Imagine a supercomputer in your heart with two buttons on it. Bring your mind's eye to what you want to eliminate. See a big, red delete button. Push that button to delete that impression, thought, energy, or emotion. Visualize what you want to create — an impression, a thought, or a feeling. Now push the big, black save button, and see the image frozen on the computer screen. The computer downloads, or imprints, this image in your heart, and it is transfers into your bloodstream through the heart's pumping. This image is broken down into countless particles, and your bloodstream distributes them throughout your body.

Here's an example. Open your hands and say, "I bring the energy of this creation I saved into my hands, my third eye, my navel, and my feet." You will feel pulsing energies there. You are circulating your intention throughout your body. When something happens inside your body, change happens outside. How do you feel, my dearest brother?

It's pretty amazing. I mean, I did what you said, and I could feel heightened energy activation in my third eye and navel — all the places you mentioned. I think time is going to tell how effective that was. I probably have to do it a few times.

Work with this for a few days, and you will feel energy pulse throughout your body. Hold this energy, and ground it into the earth. You will see. Your intention is in your body, and through your body, you implant it into Mother Earth. Everything comes from Mother Earth, but it must first happen inside your physical body before it will fully manifest into Mother Earth's body. You will be amazed at the results. When you work with it, when you go back to the supercomputer in your heart, many things can happen.

Will this work for different issues?

Yes, for different issues, but we encourage you to work with one thing at a time, and then you will see the difference, especially regarding health issues and blockages that prevent you from moving forward in life. Everything can be shifted because at a deep level, things are blocked, and these blocks manifest in a different reality.

When you are able to shift these energies, especially in your mind and your body, shifts happen naturally. We do not want to talk too much about the heart because so much has been written about it. We would just like you to practice this understanding of the supercomputer in the heart and understand the potential to change through this work.

Get in touch with the twenty-fourth chamber of your heart. Come to this place daily to feel rejuvenated and supported. Remember it contains your divine presence.

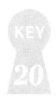

Increase Inner Light

The Family of God

Family of God: We will now talk about ascension key 20 — increasing your inner light through rhythms and patterns. Rhythms are important indicators of changes in your life. As you observe nature, you might notice that everything happens through rhythms. A seed is planted in the ground. At the appropriate time, it sprouts life. It becomes a tiny plant. Then it grows into a small shrub or a tree. Nature works in rhythmic patterns.

The pumping of blood through your body also happens rhythmically. It does not happen haphazardly. The heart of a person in good health beats in a rhythmic pattern. If the heartbeat is irregular — slower and faster — then it is time to see a doctor.

Everything has a tempo. As humans grow, there is a rhythm. At a certain time, a child will begin crawling. Then the child will put one foot in front of the other and start walking, and after some time, the child will run. Everything happens in rhythms.

Rhythms can be manipulated through your thinking. As you focus on your heart, your heart beats rhythmically. Through intention, you can cause your heart to beat faster. The same is true for breathing. There is a rhythm to your breathing, but your thoughts affect your breathing, and your emotions do as well.

Rhythms can be adjusted and manipulated to create higher frequencies. One of the rhythms is light coursing through your physical body. Light courses through every human body, but the rhythm is very faint in most people because they have not paid attention to the rhythm of light. As you focus on it, you can increase this rhythmic pattern.

Here is an example. Open the fingers of your right hand. You might not feel anything, or you might feel some energy. Focus on your right hand, and say, "I give the intention to experience the rhythmic energy in my right hand now."

I give the intention to experience the rhythmic energy in my right hand now.

You will immediately feel something in your hands, like energy. Can you feel something in your hands?

Yes. It's not what I expected. It feels like a substance, like something is there.

Something is there, but now you can ask to increase its velocity. Repeat the statement: "I give intention to experience the rhythmic patterns in my hands right now."

I give intention to experience the rhythmic patterns in my hands right now.

Make the sound "oh, oh, oh, oh."

Oh, oh, oh, oh.

Continue making the sound for about 60 seconds.

[Makes sound for 60 seconds.]

When you make this sound, you will notice the rhythm's intensity increasing.

It is doing that.

Can you feel it lighten up?

Yes. It is lightening up with the sound. It is like I am manifesting this thing in my hand to vibrate with this sound.

You can rhythmically adjust the light moving in your physical body. It is the same principle. Imagine the beautiful scene when a baby is born. Everyone says, "He's such a cute baby." They notice the sparkle in the baby's eyes. The baby is emitting light. People want to hug babies. That is love. So light exists within us always. But because we do not see the light, we do not think of it. Since people do not focus on the light, their lights do not burn outwardly. It is dimmed and slight, but now you can activate your light.

Reset Your Inner Rhythms

Light is in every place in your body, but there are places where it is more concentrated. These are called light packets. Some of these packets are beneath the sternum, not at the center of the sternum, but on both sides, near your rib cage, basically beneath your breasts. These are very important places.

We ask you to open both hands, and place your right palm in front of this place on the right side, and the left palm on the left side, beneath your breasts, and listen. Close your eyes, and be in this space. Make the sound "ho, ho, ho, ho."

Ho, ho, ho, ho.

Continue. You will feel energy in your hands.

I do.

You will feel as if you're going down inside.

It activates this area. Ho, ho, ho. [Repeats for 30 seconds.]

You will feel this energy in both hands.

I am also feeling energy in my ribs.

You are increasing the rhythmic pattern of light inside you so that it can come out.

Funny thing, I am getting visions. I don't know whether it's mental or not, but I'm get-ting visions of the house that I lived in as an infant. It was my grandmother's house in Washington.

This is not mental. This is a natural part of the exercise. You will feel tingling, as if something is moving up. This is best done for 3 minutes. You have to build the sound. Your hands will feel the energy moving.

There is a feeling of being cared for and protected.

You come back to yourself now, and more and more light is within you. You will feel more alive. You are all love. This is a really important place that calls forth light in a concentrated form.

Now, place your hands where your hips and your thighs join. This is called the psoas muscle. It is an important place because there is DNA there. Bring your hand there as you sit down, and make the sound "mooo."

Mooo, mooo. [Repeats "mooo" several times.] It is electrifying this area.

Let's continue this for 60 seconds. Make the sound deeper.

It feels like — I'm not sure what to call it — nerve impulses or something going down through my thighs.

Exactly. This is called activating the fire codes. This is a lightning code, and you will feel the energy deeply. Place your hands on top of both kneecaps [figure 20.1], and make the sound "taay, taay, taay."

Taay, taay, taay. [Repeats "taay" several times.]

You will feel that you're going deeper into solid ground.

Well, it feels just like what you said, being grounded. It feels like being really grounded to the earth.

Also, you feel that you're becoming heavier and going deeper inside. The next place is your ankles. Sit as if doing the lotus pose (yoga). Use the index and middle fingers of both hands. These fingers do not touch each other. They make a V. The ring finger and the pinkie fingers are folded and touch the middle of your palms. And the thumbs rest on them. You have two V's pointed toward the back of your ankles [figure 20.2]. Make the sound "sarrr." You can do this sitting down.

[Repeats "sarr" several times.]

It is best to do this when you're sitting on a chair with both feet down, but you could also do this sitting in a cross-legged position on the floor — however you feel comfortable.

It is very grounding. That's what I feel.

Next, cup the fingers of both hands, and touch the bottom of your spinal column. Your fingers are touching each other. Your right hand is on your right hip bone, and your left hand is on your left hip bone. [figure 20.3] This is a place of continuous energy. Make the sound "wom." Please be careful when you do this. It can be like a volcanic eruption of light, like a boom.

[Repeats "wom" several times.]

You might feel a burst of energy. Continue this for 30 seconds.

This is slower to act, but it is finally waking up back there.

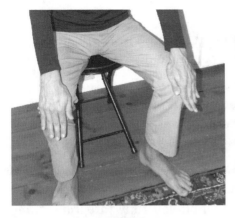

Figure 20.1

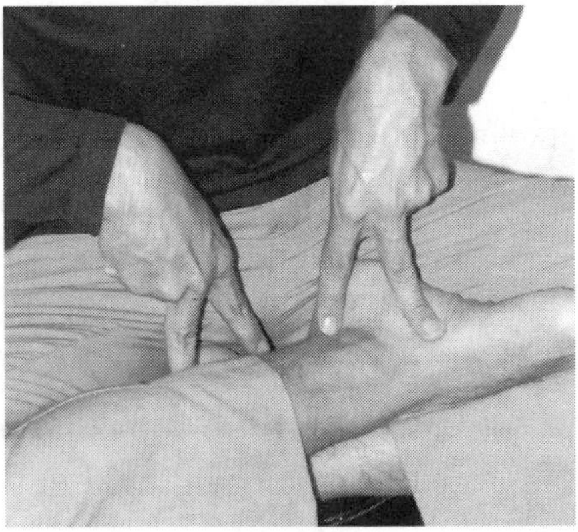

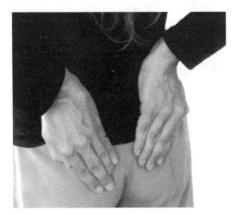

Figure 20.2

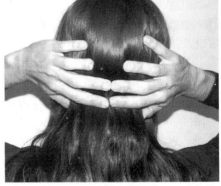

Figure 20.3

Figure 20.4

Figures 20.1–20.4. Mudras to activate fire codes

Do it, perhaps, six more times.

It's doing it, but it's slow.

Once you start moving, you will feel the most progress there and experience incredible light.

The next area is very important. This is around the middle of the medulla oblongata. Place both hands on the back of your head, the right hand on the right side and the left hand on the left side. Open all the fingers of both hands, touching the area of the medulla oblongata. The fingers are splayed, but only the middle fingers touch each other at the back of the head [figure 20.4].

Focus your attention there, and we will make a simple sound. The energy will be very soft and beautiful. This sound is "haarau." You will feel a beautiful expansion with light coming out.

[Repeats "haarau" several times.] Yes, I can see it.

It is like a curtain has been opened. Your body might shake a little bit, or it might move. You might see a night sky, blackness.

I do, and I also see ancient temples, like I'm doing this in a temple somewhere.

That is beautiful. You can put your hands down now. When you activate these points of light in you, you are increasing your rhythms of light. The beauty of this is that when you fully integrate it and reset the rhythms within you, you will be in alignment with planetary rhythms and Earth's rhythms — the Schumann resonance of Earth. You have opened and realigned the rhythms within your body to be in alignment with Earth rhythms. Everything in nature is aligned to these planetary rhythms. Now you have joined that club.

Your music is very beautiful because you are not playing solo anymore. You are becoming part of the great artistry. You are creating and cocreating energies and ideas that match everything around you. You are in the flow.

Open to
New Truths
and Realities

The Family of God

Family of God: Hello, brother. This is the Family of God. We embrace you, your home, and all the beings in your home, including the mice, the cats, the flies, the butterflies, and the trees — everything.

Thank you.

We send love to you. Today we have a big entourage, almost 13,000 spirit beings. They are waiting to hear our dialogue, for the word has gotten around.

Wow. I guess so.

This is interesting information. Today we talk about ascension key 21 — two very important parts of the physical body, the medulla oblongata and the pineal gland. The pineal gland is a spiritual gland. It regulates the movements of your physical body that regulates eye coordination and the rhythm of your heart. It is not just a spiritual gland; it is the driver of the engine. For example, a train conductor can move the train to the left track, the straight track, or the right track. It is similar to the pineal gland. It helps you to move forward, whether you are sleeping or awake. It supports your journey in life.

Have you wondered how you are able to walk? You rarely think about things like that — how a person is able to put one foot in front of the other. What gives the command at that level? The pineal gland gives the commands for everything.

It works in conjunction with the brain in that respect.

The driver of your body gives commands, and the other parts follow the commands. This is why it is called the seat of the soul. For example, suppose you cut your hand. Perhaps you were cutting vegetables, and now you are bleeding. After some time, the blood stops flowing. What directs the flow, and what causes it to stop?

Well, I think you are going to say the pineal gland. That is a guess.

Because it is the big boss.

Scientists would say that blood coagulates.

But there is a force that makes that happen, and it makes the heart beat. There is a force that creates all the rhythms of the body, even that makes the eyes twitch. Have you ever wondered how someone sneezes? Of course, there is a scientific explanation.

These are really descriptions of what happens, for the most part, not explanations.

Exactly. The pineal gland is what regulates everything. It creates rhythms and patterns, everything in the body, so that the body can function as best it can.

The pineal gland is a protein. There are many energies in the pineal gland. This is what is not really understood. The pineal gland also contains the original cell through which you were created — the joining of the seed and the ovum to create the soul where life started. This is also located in the pineal gland.

Is this the same as the signature cell?

You can call it that name, or you can call it the omega cell or the point one cell. There are different names. There are spirit beings inside the pineal gland, and the spirit beings are not masters. They are beings whose sustenance — the texture and material — created your soul. These beings live within the pineal gland because this is their home. They were used to create your soul. This is important to remember.

It's really profound.

What constitutes your soul? People say it is light and energy. Yes, it is true, but light contains frequency, and what does frequency contain? Electrons and atoms. What does an atom contain? There is a knowingness, a beingness, inside each atom, and each atom knows.

The Three Energies of the Pineal Gland

The energies of three beings are inside the pineal gland. One is the energy of Archangel Michael. One is the energy we call Imut, of which the goddesses Mother Mary and Isis are parts. "Imut" means mother. Your loving, nurturing aspect opens up because of this being. Because of Archangel Michael's energy, you have the courage to be born and face life. You might not have heard the name of the third energy in the pineal gland, for it is a being from a far-off universe. The name of this being is Gqcyriwi [pronounced "gwee"]. Your soul essence is made up of these materials, and these energies exist in your pineal gland.

Could you describe the third energy, Gqcyriwi, in more detail?

This being is from another universe. Earth is part of this universe, but there are also other universes, and we, the Family of God of this universe, interact and communicate with the creators of other universes. This spirit Gqcyriwi is from another universe, almost 230 billion light-years away.

Is it fair to describe other universes as different dimensions? I'm having a hard time conceptualizing what you mean, and a light-year seems very physical.

You could simply say it is another reality, a completely benevolent reality. Inside the pineal gland, you have three beings. When you want to get in touch with these beings, focus on your pineal gland. You will be able to perceive these energies very clearly.

Connect with Imut

Here is an exercise: Close your eyes, and open your hands so that all your fingers are splayed. Now touch your palms with the fingers of the right hand pointing up and the fingers of the left hand pointing forward [figure 21.1].

The two hands are at 90 degree angles?

Yes. All fingers are opened. Breathe into that. You will be quickly taken to another reality in a semitrance state.

It feels as if I'm going somewhere, as if I'm being transported.

Exactly. Now just stay there for a moment. When you make this hand gesture, you are communicating with the energy of Imut, the goddess. Now shake your hands.

Connect with Gqcyriwi

All fingers of your left hand are extended and closed so that there are no gaps between the fingers, including the thumb. This hand is held horizontal to the stomach, palm up. Now extend the fingers of your right hand. Touch your right elbow to the middle of your left palm. The right elbow is bent at 90 degrees, and it is held vertically, the hand pointing upward [figure 21.2]. This mudra is more powerful when you are standing. Doing this for 5 to 10 minutes can be equal to 10 hours of meditation. Do this, and immediately you will feel you are channeling us.

Yes. I feel surges of energy running down through my body.

Hold this for 60 seconds. Can you feel the stillness grow?

Yes, I do. It feels as if I'm in two places at once. Part of me is here, but part of me went somewhere else.

This is the place where Master Yeshua exists all the time. This is the place of the energy of Gqcyriwi. It is still.

Yes, there is stillness here. It is beautiful.

That is what Yeshua said. Be still. Come to this place of stillness, and you will discover yourself. Conquer the place of stillness, and discover the calm.

I can feel my heart opening to this in a very unusual way.

Now shake your hands loose. We'll do the third one.

Connect with Archangel Michael

Cup your left hand. All fingers touch each other. Hold it in front of your heart. Extend the fingers of your right hand. The right pinky and thumb touch each other. Hold your right hand next to your left hand [figure 21.3]. The three fingers of the right hand are horizontal

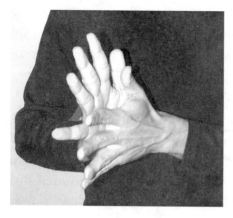

Figure 21.1

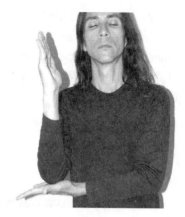

Figure 21.2

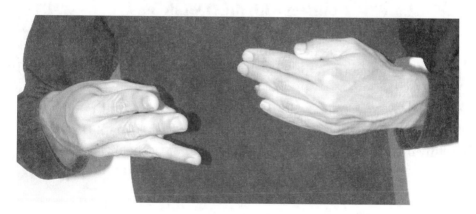

Figure 21.3

Figures 21.1–21.3. Mudras to open to new realities

to the floor. This connects you with the energy of Archangel Michael, which represents opening to new realities. Hold this position for 60 seconds. How do you feel?

Well, it's quite interesting. I would say that my glimpse here is the courage to experience.

Exactly. Why is this important? As we have learned, everything created must grow in consciousness and evolve. For that to happen, you must be willing and open to new truths.

Yes. The motivating factor here is through Archangel Michael in the pineal gland — to experience this rather than, let's say, live in the tropics and pick fruit off the trees.

Exactly — to be open to new truths, new realities. This is how we accept new realities and evolve. Life by its nature, God by nature, means evolution. It is called conscious expansion. Archangel Michael brings peace and the energy of conscious expansion from moment to moment. This energy is in the pineal gland. It is beautiful. With these hand gestures, you can connect with these masters.

So Yeshua comes from a dimension or galaxy 230 billion light-years away? That's amazing.

That's why he is considered a master. Why do you think his influence is so big? You must remember that it is not just here on Earth. His influence is extensive. It extends to the intergalactic regions and many other planets. The beings who live in those dimensions are well aware of Yeshua.

Connect with the DNA Beings in Your Pineal Gland and Medulla Oblongata

This exercise can be found on **TRACK 5, DISC 2** of the included CDs.

There are DNA beings in another reality inside your medulla oblongata and the pineal gland. They are shaped like the lotus petals, and their color is soft beige.

1. Focus on this part of your body. Breathe into it, and say, "I request the DNA beings to activate the dormant DNA within my medulla and to open the DNA within my pineal gland." As they open, you will feel faint sensations and hear sounds and chanting. Things will start spinning.

2. There are paintings from ancient Egypt depicting pharaohs with four lotus petals on the backs of their heads. As you breathe, the petals spin in harmony. They look like many petals because they are moving very fast.

3. You cannot see the individual petals clearly. They look like many slender beige leaves 6 or 8 inches long. They rotate clockwise as you look at your head from the outside. Bring your attention to this area.

4. Close your eyes, and say, "I am requesting the spirit of DNA located within my pineal gland to open the dormant energies contained in my DNA and reveal his energy to me now so that I can experience this energy." Focus your attention on this part of your body, breathe, and make the sound "zuummmmm, zuummmmm." Breathe. You will see these petals spinning as you tone "zuummmmm, zuummmmm."

5. Two things will happen: The petals will spin faster, and the lotus will open more. Then you will see light shooting upward from the petals. This is in the back of your head, like a tube of light.

6. You will see the lotus open up as you continue toning "zuumm-mmm, zuummmmm, zuummmmm." You will see a tube of light on your left extend above your head. How do you feel?

This was interesting, because at the beginning, there was some resistance. My head was turning involuntarily, but I feel incredibly nurtured now, expanded. It's quite amazing.

Of course. Of course. You are accessing the light within you.

It feels good.

7. "Zuummmmm, zuummmmm, zuummmmm." Now, from the exterior, the light goes all the way to the top of your head. Imagine, breathe, and focus on this light in front of your heart. You are directing a certain part of the light in front of your heart.

8. The light flows from the pineal gland and the medulla oblongata to above your head. From there, a portion flows to the front of your heart and then back to your pineal gland, creating a triangle. Do this for 60 seconds while toning "zuummmmm."

9. At the point of the triangle in the heart area, a door opens. It is a beautiful doorway full of light. Inside the door, you can see two intersecting circles, a vesica piscis. This is the place of Father/Mother God.

Part of me wants to cry. It is incredibly touching.

10. Look up, and say, "I request that all my meridians be connected to the vesica piscis inside the opening of my heart." The vesica piscis represents the energy of Father/Mother God within you. When you plug your meridians to this point in your body, the meridians suck the energy of Father/Mother God. The meridians will distribute this energy to all parts of your body. What you are doing is putting meridian pumps in the well of Father/Mother God, and the meridians suck this energy. The energy is a beautiful gold color, and the meridians grow throughout your body, distributing the energy of Father/Mother God all over you.

All I can say is that this is touching something very, very deep within me.

11. Of course. You are opening the medulla oblongata. There is light in the back of your head, there is light on top of your head, and there is light in front of your heart. You are inside your heart, and the meridians are plugged into the vesica piscis there. Every

moment, you are plugged into the energy of Father/Mother God. You carry this energy throughout your being. This is called living Father/Mother God from moment to moment.

12. This is the sustenance for your soul and your physical body. You are drinking liquid manna — the food of Father/Mother God. Breathe it in.

13. Make this statement silently: "This is my truth. I am Father/ Mother God, and I nourish my body, my mind, and my soul with manna, with the food of Father/Mother God." Breathe it in. Breathe it in. Breathe it in. How do you feel?

It's beautiful. I mean, words don't work here.

We will stop at this time. Do you have any questions?

I don't. This is one of the most amazing experiences I have ever had. I don't need to ask questions.

These are the new tools. You can see for yourself. In a matter of minutes, you are able to enter profound energies. Is this right?

No question.

This is a very advanced technique. It's the instant connection to higher frequencies of light.

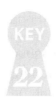

Connect with the Breath

Master Rumi

Master Rumi: Hello, dear brother. This is Master Rumi. We honor you and the land of America. It is a very special land. Although things look bleak now, there is potential for things to regenerate and for the people to unite as a nation once again. We are all very grateful for America. We love you, and we love its people.

Much has been written about the breath, so we will not go into detail. There are different kinds of breathing, and we are going to share ascension key 22 —the infinity breath technique.

You use only your right hand for this exercise. Make a fist with your right hand. All your fingers are closed except the pinky finger, which is extended. The thumb is placed over your index finger. Bring the pinky finger in front of your nose, not touching. Draw a circle in a counterclockwise [as you see it] motion. You might feel some sensations there. This helps you open to higher sensations, and it can regulate your breath.

When you regulate your breath, you can extend your breathing to anything you want and draw its energy back to you through your breath. Here is an example: Visualize Mount Rushmore with the four presidents. Breathe into the mountain and see your breath come back to your nose in an infinity symbol. Do this for 30 seconds. How do you feel, my brother?

Well, this might sound farfetched, but I feel like I am drawing on the consciousnesses of the four men who are up there.

Why do you think it's farfetched?

Well, I guess it sounds somewhat strange.

We have just given you a new tool. Close your eyes again, and breathe. Bring your attention to your breath. Point your pinky finger toward your nose as previously described, and then put your hand down at your side. Visualize a great humpback whale in the Pacific Ocean. It is splashing. It is having a great time. Its tail rises from the water. See the energy come back to you from the humpback whale in an infinity symbol.

Well, it's pretty amazing. I'm not going to say it is farfetched this time.

Can you feel it?

Oh, it's profound. I don't know what the word is, but it's great — huge depth and wisdom.

We are trying to show you that you can extend yourself to anything through your breath. I will give you another example. Close your eyes, and as you breathe normally, imagine the full moon. It is a bright, beautiful full moon. Breathe into the Moon, and feel the energy coming from the Moon to you. You will be amazed. Do this for 30 seconds. How do you feel?

Well, there's part of me that's resisting this, and it's because of things that I read about the Moon being an artificial structure that has aliens and so forth.

It's okay. What we are saying is you will be able to draw that energy to you. It can be a tree, a boat, a bird, or a goat. Just breathe. Breathe from your heart. Pay attention to your heart, and breathe your natural breath.

Visualize a golden eagle flying. It is a magnificent being, soaring above with incredible beauty. Breathe into this golden eagle, and feel its energy come into you.

It doesn't take very long. It is a very noble being.

Exactly. He is the king of birds.

He is reigning over his territory.

Good. We encourage you to do this in your meditations. When people are ready to do this exercise, they can breathe in the energy of the I Am presence, their twin flames. Close your eyes. You don't have to think of anything. Simply say, "I breathe in the energy of my I Am presence."

I breathe in the energy of my I Am presence.

You will be amazed. You might feel a shiver go through you and a downloading of energy as your whole body shakes. That can happen.

I'm not shaking, but it feels incredibly supportive and familiar to me.

Do you feel a little bit of expansion?

Oh, yes, very expanded.

Just imagine what could happen when you do this daily.

Well, I can see it would be very uplifting and transformative.

Exactly. When you do this, you bring your higher self into you, and during that time, your soul fragments naturally come back to you.

In other words, parts of my consciousness that have separated through trauma?

Yes, exactly. You are now achieving two things: returning soul fragments and integrating your I Am presence.

I will show you another thing. Close your eyes, and focus your mind's eye on Machu Picchu. Breathe into this sacred structure. Breathe into it. The journey will be amazing. How do you feel, brother?

The impressions I get from this are sacredness and ceremony, great sacredness.

You will attune to certain powers and forces in the world. You pick up many powers from Mount Shasta, Arkansas, Sedona, and certain parts of Hawaii — places all over the world. Instead of going there, you can bring their energies into you through breathing.

Now, visualize the image of a crop circle. Breathe into the crop circle. You will see the energy of the crop circle come into you.

I am having a hard time getting a reading on it. I don't know why that is. Maybe I'm not seeing a specific crop circle.

That's okay. We encourage you to do this exercise. You can pick sacred geometric patterns, sacred places, or crop circles. New crop circles are powerful energy centers, and you can connect with them.

Connect with Creation

Here is another exercise: Ask to breathe into the original intention, the coded energy of Gaia, before Gaia was set up to be a planet for human beings. Ask to speak to the beings who created this. When you do this exercise, in less than three months, you will start channeling these beings because these beings will become part of you. They are ready to be channeled.

For example, you felt the consciousness of the Founding Fathers on Mount Rushmore. Imagine you have done this exercise for a few days. What will happen? Their consciousnesses and your consciousness will combine, and when someone asks you a question, the answer will come from this joint consciousness. You will be channeling these beings. Do you see?

Yes, I do. It's quite amazing.

You are taking on or becoming acquainted with their vibration without taking on the whole consciousness.

You do not go anywhere. You sit in your living room and extend yourself to these places and the energy through your breath.

This brings up the energetic connection. When you do this infinity loop, you will be taking on only benevolent energies.

Okay, so that's the screen. That's the filter.

This must be done in order. The techniques in this book must be done in the order given. You can also breathe the twelve planets or your astrological sign. Here is an example. Close your eyes and become one with the planet. Let's start with Saturn. Say, "I breathe into Saturn," and imagine your breath going to Saturn and coming back to you in an infinity loop pattern as you breathe. How do you feel, my brother?

Well, I can feel it, but it's hard to put it into words.

Yes. Now, we ask you to do an experiment. Write down the names of the twelve planets [to refer to during this breathing exercise], and then breathe into each planet. When these planetary energies are integrated within you, you will become balanced with all twelve planets.

Do you do them separately first?

Yes, you will see a very subtle difference between each planet's energy in you. You can also do this with stars, such as the Pleiades or Arcturus. When you do this, you integrate high frequencies of light from these higher beings. These energies are spirit beings, and naturally your light quotient goes up incredibly. You will also start channeling these beings, which simply means you are becoming one with all creation. This is called "I am in communion with all creation." Is this not beautiful?

It is beautiful.

Connect with Yeshua

Are you ready for the magic now?

It's been pretty magical so far.

Okay, close your eyes. Visualize the image of Master Yeshua. Perhaps he's carrying a sheep in his hand. He's wearing a beautiful white coat. He has a beard and a beautiful, kind face. Breathe into this incredible master. How do you feel, brother?

Wow! It's amazing. I mean, I can feel his consciousness.

If you do this for 5 minutes, you will cry.

I almost cried here.

The tears will come, such love. You are becoming one with the consciousness of Yeshua. That means there is no separation. Do this simple method. You will slowly realize you are one with all creation, and there has never been separation. It was just an illusion. You can use simple breathing techniques to transform, understand, and experience this new reality.

You can do this with mountains. You can do this with water. We encourage you to connect with the four elements. Connect with the spirit of the forest and the jungles. Connect with whales and dolphins. Connect with the energy of butterflies, deer, alpaca, golden eagles, black bear, grizzly bear, kangaroos, and penguins. Connect with the twelve planets, the planet Kepler-48, and rainbows.

You will feel close to all creation through this exercise. Your vision will expand. Your mind will expand. You will have love coming into you from all these things.

You can extend to any masters you want to connect with. You can connect with your ancestors. You can say, "Who was Robert's great-great grandfather?" Then breathe into him, and send your balanced energy into him in the past. This can heal people. Because you are your ancestors and you carry the energy of your ancestors in you, you heal yourself and your ancestral past. You also heal your ancestral being. Enjoy the breath work.

• • •

I am Rumi. This book contains profound and simple methods. When you are committed to this, you will see how this simple infinity breath technique supports the integration of higher light.

ℛestore ℱood's
𝒪riginal ℰnergy

Gaia

Gaia: Hello, dear brothers, Robert and Rae. Thank you for the opportunity to bring forth a new understanding about your role on Earth to help you more quickly attain what you have been seeking throughout your lives and through many incarnations. Today we will talk about ascension key 23 — restoring your food's energy.

Food plays a vital role in humanity's awakening. Many of you bless your food, but food can also be programmed. You might ask, "How can I program my food? I do not have control over it." Perhaps you are eating at a restaurant or purchasing food at the supermarket. Whatever the case, you can send a thought projection from your heart to the food. Visualize a vegetable or fruit in its original form before it was harvested. This might take 10 or 15 seconds. Hold the intention for this food to replenish your health. The energy goes where your thoughts go. When you open your heart, you send energy laced with golden light to the fruit, vegetable, or other food you want to eat.

Beaming this energy from your heart awakens the very essence of the food, which might have been subdued or lost in the process of harvesting, freezing, or transporting. This means that the vegetable will carry its original energy once again. Thus, when you eat this food, you take in its original content and energy.

You will notice that you will eat less because your food will have more of its original energy, which is the energy of pure love. A small portion will fill your stomach. This will take some time to practice, but you will be amazed at the results. You are energetically programming your food!

Let's say you're eating bread or a bagel. It is made from many ingredients. Visualize the ingredients in their original forms. You might not be able to do this with every ingredient, but visualize them as best you can for 10 seconds. Then open you heart to each one, and send that energy to the food. That's all. You've programmed your food.

For example, you purchased an avocado. You can visualize the avocado on a tree with many other avocados. They are happy and healthy, and a gentle breeze is blowing. The avocado feels happy, and when you eat it, you eat the avocado's spirit, and you are happy as well. Eating avocados will increase your brain capacity exponentially, and the juice of an avocado can condition your heart. Your kidneys can be adjusted to function properly. Focus on the intention you want this food to accomplish in your body. This is how the masters did it.

Support for Ascension

The old yogis and masters ate very little. They programmed their food so that it gave them the life force they needed to nourish the different parts of their bodies. You can ask the spirit of your food to support the awakening or health of any part of your body. For example, you can ask for compassion to fill your heart. Tomatoes are especially good for this, particularly small tomatoes.

You can communicate your intention to your fruit and vegetables, and they will do the work because they carry pure energy. Just imagine what this could do for your physical body when practiced regularly. Many sicknesses can be changed or alleviated. If your organs are damaged, they could be healed — perhaps not fully, but you will see a shift. This depends on your belief system and how long you work at it.

We encourage you to follow this simple exercise. Hold the intention for the food you eat to support the integration of all higher life from all dimensions so that you can ascend and join with your life force again. You will be in complete harmony and cooperation with you food. You can do this with all food. Then your food becomes your best friend.

. . .

You have certainly heard the expression "you are what you eat." Now you will be more conscious of what you eat. Your body, mind, and spirit will be pleased and able to support your destiny. This is a short message, but we believe it is powerful. It can shift your life if you work at it.

Ignite Creation Energies

Spirit of Fire

Spirit of Fire: Many people are afraid of me. They see fire as dangerous, that it can kill. Fire is as a knife in that it can be used for many purposes. Without fire, there is no life. Today we will discuss ascension key 24 — the element of fire and how it creates energy for you to survive. Fire is connected to the first ray of God. It is also connected to the magnificent energy of Archangel Michael and the great golden eagle. All represent the incredible powers of the human soul. You can work with fire gently and direct it.

Fire is the spark within your life. It is the creative input, the zest for living, the enthusiasm, and the cheerfulness. Fire can also be used for a higher purpose. There are chakras in your physical body that convey many frequencies of light. There are healing chakras, karmic chakras, and fertility chakras. These are important in different ways.

You can program fire and communicate with it to clear the dross of the energy embedded in the tissues and cells of your physical body. Your body can only burn away so much of these heavy, dense energies. There are many dense energies in your organs, tissues, hair, skin, nails, and other places in your body. You can bring the energy of fire to these places to clear out all the dross or worn-out energy with the power of your mind. However, you must be careful because fire can be deadly. If you use too much, it can do damage.

Bringing fire to your body is important, especially for elderly people. It reinvigorates them, returning enthusiasm to their lives. As people retire from their work, most are still in good shape. When they lose their work routines, they often spend more time being idle, such as watching television. Their bodies sag from the lack of activity, and they feel tired. They are not fully participating in life anymore. Bring the energy of fire to them. Simply breathe it into them. Do this through the small toes.

There are chakras beneath the nails of the four small toes on both feet. Brother Robert, bring your attention to the small toes beneath the toenails. These chakras are orange and shaped like a small spiral. Imagine a small spiral there, and breathe into them. You can make the sound "oram."

Oram, oram, oram, oram.

You'll start feeling energies in your toes.

It feels like energy is being drawn into my foot through my toes.

Then this energy will move up through your body.

That's right; it is going up.

When you do this for 5 or 6 minutes regularly, this energy will spread through your body and regenerate your cells. It will burn away many of the heavy, dense energies there. When this energy dissipates, minute particles of light embedded in your cells will open up. This is like digging for gem stones. You have to remove the topsoil, and then you will find a beautiful gem. Done regularly, this simple exercise can help you understand your life's purpose because you will cleanse yourself with fire energy.

Do this gently and slowly and not for more than 5 or 6 minutes each day. That's all. You will become lighter. Your kundalini is powered by fire, and it will rise gently and automatically without doing anything additionally.

Many people who want to awaken very quickly will overdo it, and if they are not ready, their organs can be damaged by the high intensity of fire. It can also play tricks on their minds. All that is needed is about 5 or 6 minutes each day. This is best done early in the morning. Avoid doing it at night because it can disrupt sleep.

When people overdo it, they might feel hot, irritated, and restless. They might move around and not get anything done because their minds are not at peace. They could feel unfocused. They might also become angry or irritated much more quickly than usual. They could behave aggressively. These are all signs that there's too much fire in them.

Ground the Fire Energy

Fire can be anchored in the earth. Once you feel the energy in your toes, try sending it into the ground. This will help heal the land. There are many dark energies embedded in the ground as soul imprints — things like fear and hatefulness. They are all embedded in the ground and can be healed.

When people die, their strongest emotions, feelings, and beliefs are imprinted on their souls. People return with strong soul imprints. These can be shaped. You can ask for this during your meditations by saying, "I call the Spirit of Fire and Master Sananda to guide me and help me so that I can use the Spirit of Fire to transmute soul imprints I have carried from other lifetimes, especially the soul imprints of lack, the belief that life is a struggle and that I will always be poor, the feeling that life is without purpose, and feelings of unworthiness." Ask the heavy-duty soul imprints to be transmuted by the Spirit of Fire.

You will feel a shift in about fifteen days, but remember that some soul imprints will not be removed because they are part of your karmic lesson in this lifetime. Many other belief systems and smaller soul imprints can be released.

Thank you. This was very helpful.

Work with your toes every day, and make the sound "oram."

Thank you.

Shift Consciousness Energy

Gaia

Gaia: Hello, family. This is Gaia. We thank you for the opportunity to speak to our brothers and sisters through this medium. We are going to discuss ascension key 25 — changing the density of water.

Water has many structures and different densities depending on where it comes from. For example, the water in a brook at the base of a mountain is low in density. This is why people feel good near a brook or a waterfall. They feel welcome to put their feet or their hands in the water. Water of this density contains a certain consciousness.

The Nile River is an example of dense water. It starts in East Africa, and it runs through many countries until it comes to Egypt. It supports the people of Egypt, but the water is very dense there. Egypt is still struggling. There is much poverty and suffering. In India, there are many sacred, holy rivers, but the water is not as pure in the plains as it was at the beginning of the river. It flows through many territories and states, and it affects people's consciousness.

Bless the Water within You

Water density varies by country, whether it is in a lake or a river. We are not talking about seawater. That was designed for a different purpose. The water in certain countries is designed for completing the karmic energy there. Certain waterways are deliberately made dense so that people can forget. Let's use Egypt as an example. Many people living on the banks of the Nile still live the same way that people lived for thousands of years. Nothing much has changed. It is the density that keeps people trapped in those patterns. It happens so that they can work out their karma.

People have pure consciousness, so they can work out their karma. This is not generally understood by humanity. People must change the density of the water that exists in their country through prayers and meditations. They need to send loving energy from their hearts into the waterways, and then the water will shift in density. People will also shift in exactly the right proportion. Let's look at Vietnam. There is change in Vietnam, but the waterways are quite dense, and the rivers run through the middle of the cities. However, the country is moving forward. In what way is it moving forward?

It sounds to me that you're saying this may not be the ideal way to move forward. Is that correct?

Yes, exactly. There is a tendency to be in the world to make money as fast as you can, but people can forget the bigger picture. When water is very clear and it flows through cities where people live, you will see a crack, an opening, to higher consciousness and higher truth.

Bless any liquid you take into you to change its molecules and its density. When you bless something, you shift its energies. When you drink blessed water, you change the density of the water inside you, and you naturally awaken to higher consciousness. So bless the water within you every day. Ask your bone marrow to produce less density and clearer, lighter water. Your bones will acknowledge you when you make your request.

When you drink any sort of liquid, ask to change the density of the water to light. This light goes directly into your bone marrow, and the density of the water in your entire body shifts. This must be done with proper recognition of water through your feelings and through your heart.

Water is a living being. It can hear what you think. If you do this casually, it will not cooperate, but if you ask it to change, you will see much wisdom come into you, and other karmic energies will disperse. You will increase your light frequency.

Troubled people can bless all the water they drink and be converted to light through their bloodstreams. When they do this for 10 days, they will see a shift.

The steps you have outlined are for people to change the density of the water they consume. Is it too soon to think about praying for waters in rivers and larger areas?

We want you to come to this understanding very quickly for all the waters around the world — in your country and everywhere. When you pray for the water to be shifted in a certain area, there will be a shift in people's karmic consciousness there before they access higher wisdom. Then they will change that karma.

Karma is changed through wisdom. It is not through the physical experience they are going through. Karma is changed through gaining wisdom.

Sense Higher Frequencies

Commander Ashtar

Commander Ashtar: This is Commander Ashtar. Love, blessings, and greetings to your beautiful land. It seems that Pandora's box has been opened in the United States as well as some other countries. But don't get caught up in this. You can shift, and you can stand out.

Now we talk about ascension key 26 — celestial scents. There are scents in the celestial world just as there are in the 3D world. Celestial scents originate from flames in the temple of scents. The flames emit various scents, and we encourage people to go to these temples in consciousness to partake in this. The flames emit sound frequencies, and scents are released through them. One of the scents being emitted is transmutation. This flame is a beautiful purple.

When these celestial scents come to a physical body, they are first sensed through your fingers and then through your arms, shoulders, and down through your throat to your navel. They are activated fully inside the navel. This place needs healing in almost all human beings. This is a place where people have abused their power. They have misused or underutilized it.

This energy of transmutation can be healed. Now, brother Robert, we ask you to open the fingers of your hands, and say, "I breathe in the scent of transmutation." Just breathe it in, and visualize a beautiful purple flame.

I breathe in the scent of transmutation.

As you breathe this flame, visualize it flowing into your fingertips, going up into your elbows, moving up to and down through your shoulders, passing through your throat, and settling down into your navel.

Breathe this beautiful purple flame, and see it go into your navel area. You don't have to say anything. It will naturally transmute, recalibrate, and adjust this power point — either misused or underused power. It will balance the energy there. You might see a geometric pattern. A golden needle might appear as you breathe into the purple flame.

I can feel the energy swirling around a lot, and it feels like releasing, like something is being transmuted.

This area is where the energy of misused or underused power is stored. It is underutilized because people believe they are not good enough, so they have not used their power. Other people have used their power to destroy.

When you follow this simple procedure — using the flame of transmutation and healing this area around your navel — you will experience the scents. Why is this important? When you develop this sense of smell, you will smell energies. You will be able to smell people's intentions, and you will be able to make decisions from these scents and not just from physical appearances that people show you. This means you will utilize your sense of smell more fully.

Is it fair to say that we will use the sense of smell to get a read on people's energy and intentions?

You will know people's truth and intentions. You can use your sense of smell in a supermarket. Breathe deeply, and ask whether eating the food you want to purchase will support your body. You also could sense how you feel about a person. When you use your natural senses, you use all your senses properly, and your senses do not lie. Anywhere you go, you can smell intention. If you want to know the truth about something, you can just smell. Breathe it in, and see how your body reacts.

How does this help with your ascension process? Please write "Aum" on a piece of paper, and then beneath it write "Yod-Heh-Vav-Heh (YHVH), Yahweh." This is the name of God in Hebrew. Now close your eyes and focus your attention on Aum. You don't need to make the sound. Just imagine what your nose senses from the sound. You are breathing this sound. Don't make any sound at all. Just breathe this sound. You will see energy lift from this word into your brain and into your third eye.

I can feel my third eye opening up as I do this.

Do this for about 30 seconds, and then do it for the word "Yahweh." Just breathe in the sound "Yahweh." You might see color patterns or small flames come up from the word in your third eye and go into your brain and forehead. Just breathe it in. Don't say the word. Just breathe it in. How do you feel?

Well, it's amazing, actually. I mean, I'm close to tears on the second one. It feels so profound and familiar. In some ways, I am recognizing something that I had never seen before.

What you are doing now is breathing in truth, the energy behind the words. It goes throughout your body. It touches your heart, does it not?

It has touched most of my emotions too.

Just imagine that you are able to breathe higher-frequency thoughts and higher-frequency words. You are being freed from your common sense, which is good. This is not common sense in a small way. You are releasing the natural scent to see the truth behind every word, every situation, every person, every circumstance, and every condition.

The next time you listen to music, say, "I am going to breathe in this music." You will be amazed. You will feel the very essence of the music come into you. Imagine that you hear a violin. Do not listen. Rather, breathe in the frequency emitted by the strings. Do you think that this will enhance you? I'm sure it will.

Receive God's Love

There are higher-frequency words in every language. Pick a few from your culture. Honor the Divine, and honor the mother. In India, they pick up a language that has a higher-frequency of thought. In your way, you do it also in America, and South America does it in their way. Breathe in sounds. Smell the words. Smell the frequencies. This will enhance your light very quickly.

This is how we, the Ashtar command, and other beings in this reality are able to maintain higher frequencies, because we breathe in sounds, the great central sound. Here is a sound we can give you: "ikkem."

Ikkem.

Breathe in the sound "ikkem." Something might open inside you. This word simply means, "I am ready to receive God's love today."

That's amazing. What I felt as I was breathing this was a solid platform from which everything grows — a base. It feels very solidifying.

Yes. That means you are receiving God's love. See how easy it is? Certain sounds — just breathe them. They might not be long sentences, just single words.

I will say goodbye at this time.

Thank you. That was very profound.

We thank you for sharing the God within all of us, brother. We love and honor you.

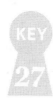

Connect with Body Numerology

Goddess Roopeshwari

Note: Do not do the exercises in this chapter before doing those in the preceding chapters. They can have a very big effect on the human psyche, and the body must prepare energy to come to this space.

Goddess Roopeshwari: Thank you for taking the time to be here so that we can bring you this information. It is not only for ascension but also for humanity's overall well-being and the planet herself. I am here to bring understanding about numbers in the human body. In nature, everything is perfect, from the tip of a bud to a tree branch to a spider's web. Everything is designed in perfection.

When human beings want to create something, they go to a drawing board. Whether they want to design a car, a house, an airplane, or a ship, they don't build it right away. Their idea begins on paper. They plan it, and then they draft it. They use mathematical and geometric patterns. The operating systems of your computer are mathematical. Mathematics and geometric patterns underlie all creation.

Humans are more complex than a ship, a leaf, or anything else.

Human beings are magnificent creations. A baby develops from a single cell into an infant. What transformation and what magic takes place from one cell to a baby! How is that possible? The process of growing a human body includes mathematics, geometry, and souls. A baby's body aligns with a particular soul.

Now we will talk about ascension key 27 — numerology of the body. Numbers are very important. Numerology is not just about finding your birth number. Numerology is much larger than that. In the future, numerology will be taught in universities because understanding numbers can help you significantly. NASA scientists work with numbers. People in financial services crunch numbers all the time. Forecasting uses numbers. Numbers play a large part in creation.

Certain numbers correspond to certain parts of the body. We'd like to give you these numbers.

The Brain — 36

The brain has the number 36 [three-six]. The 3 represents the three parts of a human being — the body, mind, and soul. The 6 represents divine sacredness with the One. These numbers are embedded in the structure of the brain.

When people ascend, their brains and thought processes shift. This is a shift in consciousness. The brain is vast. You cannot comprehend the capacity of the brain, but the shift happens inside it.

When the three join — body, mind, and soul — then the trinity is created. The 6 represents sacred divinity. Then you understand that you are a divine being: "I am the soul. I am the monad. I am the I Am presence. I Am That I Am." Isn't it beautiful, brother?

It is; it is. I'm very moved by what you're saying.

The brain holds the number 36 [three-six]. When you meditate, imagine those numbers in your brain. You will feel energy move into the brain. The 3 and 6 will join. You see how perfectly they fit together.

When the shift happens in the brain, you can experience the shift in the physical body. You are able to live your essence as a living truth. That is the meaning of life — that every little limb has spirit. Your essence is a physical truth in your physical reality. This is the meaning of 36.

The Earlobes — 42

The next number in the human body is for the earlobes, and it is 42 [four-two]: 42 means sacred divinity. The ears are as important as the eyes because there are three main chakras in the ears. When these chakras are activated, your ability to hear at a great distance is awakened.

You may have heard about the fully ascended Asian master Guanyin who can perceive the sounds of the world. He is able to pick up the sonic energy emitted by a thought. This is what animals do. Animals are able to pick up scents, thus sound frequencies, emitted by beings from great distances. Many masters are able to hear sounds that originate from very far away because the sensitivity of their ears is developed.

The Eyes — 63

Your eyes do not just take in what you see. They are sensors, and there are chakras on your eyebrows. The eyebrows are miniature sensors. The eyes see and send commands to the brain, and the brain interprets the commands, saying, "I saw 'this.'" The sensors join thoughts by the brain with the eyes. Your eyes take in a lot of energy, as much as your breath.

Blind people have developed and heightened their other senses because they do not pick up energy through their eyes. They pick up energy through other senses. Because you pick up energy through your eyes, the other senses are not used as much.

Many people who live and work in modern cities have tired eyes. The first step in Reiki to alleviate this is placing your palms over your eyes. When you relax your eyes, your whole body relaxes. You can place your hands over your eyes now. Close your eyes, cup both hands, and place them over your eyes. In a matter of seconds, you will feel warmth.

Yes, there is a transmission of energy into the eyes from the hands.

If your eyes are tired, you will feel the tired energy in your hands moving back and forth, crisscrossing. Otherwise, your eyes will start relaxing. You will feel warmth, and most people fall asleep in 8 to 10 minutes. This can help elderly people who cannot sleep.

The number for the eyes is 63 [six three]. This represents the ability to see as God sees. God sees perfection in every human being, not on the surface, but deeply within each person. God sees beauty.

You might find much ugliness in third-dimensional reality. Yes, it is true, but when you see through God's eyes, you are not only seeing this reality, you are seeing the overall reality. When you look at the whole, the lower energies are only a tiny portion.

Even a person who commits a great crime has some love in his heart — maybe love for his family or an animal. God sees the larger aspects. There is no judgment through God's eyes. You could say this person is doing something from his base instincts, but he also has higher chakras and higher energies he is not displaying because he has forgotten them.

Mother Theresa said that she would not serve the devil. She chose to serve God. Nelson Mandela forgave his oppressors and said that he chose to see God in others. This is the meaning of "namaste": "The God in me honors the God in you."

So meditate on the number 63 [six three], and focus on the eyes. Close your eyes, brother, and see 63 in your mind's eye. The 6 is a beautiful platinum color, and the 3 is a soft-pink color. Just breathe and visualize: "six three" [63].

Six-three [63].

"Six three" [63]. "Six three."

Six three [63]. Six three [63].

You might feel some heaviness in your eyes initially, so focus internally on the colors platinum and soft pink. You will also feel energy in your third eye area.

Yes, my eyes are getting heavy.

Yes, exactly, and slowly you will close your eyes and go into a deep trance state. "Six three."

Six-three [63]. Six three. It feels like if I were to continue with this, it would be like crossing a threshold into another dimension.

Exactly, into another reality. When you cleanse and deeply relax the eyes, the psychic chakras in your temples open up.

That's interesting because I can feel my temples; they feel activated.

Exactly. And they will open because of the heavy, dense energy that has gathered in your eyes. These chakras are blocked. Also, just imagine how much you see and make judgments. Look at the situation in America now, where people are so polarized. When you look closer, you see more — what someone said or did not say or why someone did something — you make value judgments. Imagine how many things you can see, such as the wars and the cruelty. But you see good things too. As you look at the world and see so much destructive energy, your eyes pick up that energy. So heal your eyes.

So the eyes absorb all the energies of discord.

Exactly. The eyes absorb the matrix energy more than anywhere else on your body. So heal your eyes with the number of 63.

The Shoulders — 14

The shoulders are next. The number for the shoulders is 14 [one four]. This means using your natural senses, the five senses that you use to experience your life. If you used your natural senses to their fullest capacity, you would not react to situations as you do now, and your life would be different. You only use 10 to 15 percent of your natural sense capacity. Things have to be observed. When you are aware, you will be able to observe and ask yourself, "How much of my sense capacity am I using now?"

Now we'd like to do an experiment, brother. Imagine your shoulders. Visualize a very shiny soft green; it has a metallic tinge. See the number 14 [one four] on each shoulder. Imagine soft-green light, like a bed of light, and on each shoulder sits the number 14 [one four]. Just breathe it in. Breathe it in. You will see the numbers move. Breathe this in. You will feel heaviness in your shoulders. The breathing combined with the numbers can help you release deep-seated karmic energies embedded in your shoulders.

Usually the shoulders carry burdens. That's been my experience when working with people.

This is because two chakras, called the karu chakras, are on the shoulders (one on each shoulder). This is why karmic energy flows into the back of the body, creating back pain. So as you said, it feels like a burden. It is a burden of the heavy, dense energies you carry.

When you work with this number, 14 [one four], you will be able to release many past beliefs and built-up energies you have carried from your ancestors. You are carrying the energy of your ancestors, the energy of their land and culture, and energy that you have created. This number can help you release that accumulated energy. Initially, you will feel heaviness on your shoulders. But later, you'll feel lightness.

I'm at the heaviness point. I'm feeling pressure on my shoulders.

Yes, initially, you will feel pressure. Eventually it will stop, and then you will see this number go deep and embed into you. It is going deeper and deeper into you. Sometimes you will feel a pain in your hands, but then they become warm and lighter. This will happen even during the first session; it can happen instantly.

Once these numbers go deep within you, the heaviness will go away. Initially, the energy is felt in your hands up to the fingers and in the shoulders, and then the hands and the shoulders will become light.

Do this exercise, and you will feel a shift. When that happens, you will release a lot of karmic energy embedded in your hands. You have used your hands along with your mouth and eyes to create karma. You use your hands to create and do everything. There is heavy-duty karma in your hands. It is possible that when you work with these numbers and your hands become lighter, old skin will come off. Your skin will feel rough and peel off, as snakes shed their skins. This means you are releasing past karmic energy. When that happens, your hands become healing hands.

That's interesting. So in other words, doing this exercise with the number 14 [one four] on the shoulders will eventually cause exfoliation, which means shedding old skin.

Exactly, exactly.

The Navel — 91

The navel is next. The number for the navel is 91 [nine one]. Your navel is the center point of your body. There is an equal length above and below your navel.

Yes, and horizontally.

Exactly, it is the center of your body. This is also the place of the sun chakra and the emotional body. Your energy is very strong in this part of the body. When you are afraid or have an anxiety attack, this place can become knotted. People say, "My stomach is in knots." It becomes very hard and emotionally tightened.

This exercise might release minor pain in this part of your body. Are you ready to try it?

Yes.

Close your eyes and see 91 [nine one] six times around your navel — 91, 91, 91, 91, 91, 91. The numbers surround your navel in a soft orange. As you breathe, they will spin, and you will feel some pain in that area.

So mine are spinning counterclockwise from my view point.

Yes. You will feel energy coming out of the numbers and going into the navel, releasing pain or heaviness. Do this for 1 minute. Breathe it in — 91, 91, 91, 91, 91, 91, 91, 91, 91, 91. You will see a geometric pattern appear around the navel.

Well, it was spinning like crazy.

You might feel some pain or discomfort.

It felt very chaotic.

Exactly, and it will continue. Some people will feel a bit nauseous. Deep cleansing, irritation, and anger can be released. Then slowly a beautiful golden pyramid will appear, and when that happens, raise the number 91 [nine one] into the pyramid. It will become a part of your reality.

So this is a cleansing or clearing technique one should use with caution?

Exactly. Doing it for 7 to 9 minutes makes it a very powerful tool. You will push out heavy energy, and you might feel uncomfortable or experience some minor pain for a couple of hours in your navel. It might not happen, but it's possible that people with heavy, dense energy might feel pain.

The Knees — 69

Next are the knees with the number 69. This number can give you the ability to have faith in your goodness and in the light you carry. This is one of the biggest problems for human beings. On a deep level, most people feel they are not worthy of the light. Even when their minds say, "I'm ready to accept the light," on a deep level, this is a test for them. Do they really doubt themselves? At the last minute, will they acknowledge that they are good enough to receive the light from God? There is so much resistance — even minor — from past lives.

When you move through that resistance, you can finally say, "I believe in my truth and in my light." Ascension is not just ascending. It is also descension. It is the light coming down to you from higher chakras. It is not that you're going up. You are bringing your higher chakras into you.

You start believing in your light. You believe in yourself deep, deep down. Can I ask you one thing? How many people accept themselves as they are at this moment?

Not very many.

Maybe they think they are too fat or too tall. It doesn't matter. People do not accept themselves 100 percent as they are. They say, "I have done bad things. I have done 'this' or 'that.' I have hurt people." On a deep level, they resist accepting those aspects of themselves. They focus on what they don't have and see it before the light that they do have, or they focus on something they did and think it was not right. They judge themselves: "Am I worthy to stand in front of God?" Just imagine if Jesus appeared in front of you. Would you accept him? Initially, you would say, "How can he appear in front of me? I am a sinner. I have done bad things." It is very difficult, brother, very, very difficult.

So when you work with your knees and anchor the energy of 69 [six nine] there, it simply means, "I accept the truth of who I am." This is one of the keys given by the god Osiris.

Do you accept that you are the truth of who you are? Are you ready to stand in your truth, brother? Work with your knees — "six nine" [69], "six-nine." See a band of platinum light flashing "69" into your knees. This is also very good for people who have knee problems.

This also means, "I can stand on my own in the world. I'm not going to run away. I am going to face my problems and solve them." It means, "I am courageous." So strengthen your knees, and you will feel courageous in your life: "six nine" [69].

The Toes — 74

Look at your toes. In many cultures, big toes represent higher wisdom in shamans. In their higher wisdom, higher love, and higher compassion, elders' toes are much bigger, and the gap between the big toe and the second toe is a little bit wider. Have you seen people's feet like that?

Yes. Is this how they're depicted artistically?

Yes, because they carry compassion and acceptance. The number is 74 [seven four]. Smile, there are chakras beneath your feet! Adding 7 and 4 [7 + 4 = 11] yields two things. The first is 11, which is the master number of a teacher. When you add 1 and 1 [1 + 1 = 2], you get 2. This represents your ability to live in the world and experience the Divine. Without physical reality, you cannot experience the Divine.

To experience the Divine, there must be a vehicle. How can you experience the absolute without the relative? The relative can be experienced in the physical reality. How do you experience it? Through your physical body.

Yes, you need something like a medium, a physical medium, to do this.

Exactly. And your legs support your physical body.

Right. So when you're speaking of the toes, you are only speaking of the two big toes, is that correct?

No, all the toes. But the two big toes have a lot of DNA in them. There are chakras on all the toes and more chakras on the bottoms of your feet. Some paintings of ancient Indian gods and of the Buddha show sacred geometric patterns beneath their feet. Have you seen pictures of sacred geometric patterns? They have DNA. So the number for toes, 74 [seven four], represents a master number (11), which means fully learning everything. You become a master teacher to others through your life because every word you say and every action you take is a definition of who you are. You walk in this knowledge of your mastery. You become very erect.

This means, "I will be good to myself, and I will be good to others." It also means, "I am beneficial to myself, and I am beneficial to others."

Some people's second toes are longer than their big toes. Is there any significance to that?

Yes, it means they have wisdom from the stars. Those people definitely have star connections.

My second toe is longer than the big toe.

Some people have six toes on one foot.

Oh, but that's very rare.

Very rare, yes, but it is important. They carry beautiful wisdom.

The Auric Body — 226

The number for the auric body is 226 [two two six]. When you add the numbers together [2 + 2 + 6 = 10], you have 10, and 1 + 0 = 1. You came from One, and there is only One, and you are part of One.

Imagine there is a ray of light encircling you, a ray of light. And there are many ones scattered in that light — 1, 1, 1, 1, 1, 1, in beautiful white light. Close your eyes. Focus on your third eye, and see 1s there. They will turn now — "one" [1].

One.

"One."

One.

"One. One. One." This will strengthen your connection to the Creator, not through any branch of religion, but to our Creator, the unidentifiable intelligence, the energy that makes everything. Your aura will also be clear, and you will feel a centeredness, a grounded-ness, and an expansion. How do you feel, brother?

Well, it's very interesting. When I was doing that, it felt as if a tube was on my third eye. If I had to describe it, it was like the center tube in a roll of paper towels extending out, and I was looking through it. It seemed that it was extending into other dimensions.

Yes, you are starting to connect directly with the source from which you were created. You became one with the Lord. You become one with the One.

I didn't do it for very long, but it seems to have the potential to expand.

The Mental Body — 313

The next number, 313 [three one three], is for the mental body. Adding these numbers [3 + 1 + 3 = 7] represents sacred experiencing, the understanding and experiencing of the sacredness of everyday life.

This number helps you to see life as a gift, not as a burden. Life is a gift through which you experience the larger part of yourselves and the Creator. You start living your lives with sacredness. You start doing things in a sacred way for yourselves and for others. You will say, "I am a sacred being." In that realization, everything shifts within you. You speak sacred words, think sacred thoughts, eat sacred food, and see with sacred eyes. Everything shifts. You come to a place of appreciation and gratitude. Jesus talked about developing the quality of gratitude.

The mind is very tricky and the shift must happen in the mind — the mental body — because the mind always focuses on what you do not have, what you desire, or what you think you need to survive. The shift must happen in the mind, but the mind will not let go. So when you work with 313 [three one three], this can happen.

Close your eyes, brother, and see the number 313 aligned vertically on top of your head, extending all the way up to your twelfth chakra. See the number 3 on the top, 1 in the middle, and 3 on the bottom. It is a pale red orange. Chant "three one three." You will see this number descend into you, and one number will go into your face, one number will go into the middle of your body, and one number will be at your feet — "three-one-three" (313).

Three-one-three (313). Three-one-three (313).

The 3 has the quality of the energy of fire. So you will see this fire energy go into you. "Three one three. Three one three." You can do it in your mind's eye. "Three one three. Three one three."

Yes, I'm doing it, and it's interesting. My whole body is starting to tingle as I do this. I feel tingling in my arms.

Close your eyes, and bring your hands into prayer position. Now chant "three one three" twelve times. You can also do this silently.

Three one three. [Chants twelve times.]

How do you feel, dear brother?

Well, I felt a number of things going on with my body. My navel area was tingling away, and my arms were tingling. It's hard to describe it all, but there were certainly a lot of things going on!

Can you feel the energy, brother?

Oh, totally. Various things were going on as we went through that.

So there will be a clearing of the mental body and the power of the mind to influence the body will start shifting.

How would it shift? Will the wisdom of the body take over?

Exactly. The mind will lose its power. The mind will still work with you but slowly, under you, not the other way around.

Yes. So it won't have a life of its own, so to speak.

Exactly.

The Emotional Body — 716

The number for the emotional body is 716 [seven one six]. When you add the numbers [7 + 1 + 6 = 14], you get 14, and 1 + 4 = 5. You experience emotions using your five senses. The number 5 also represents the ability to use the five attributes you are born with. These are discernment, responsibility, divine action, nonattachment to outcome, and stillness. When you are in this space, you become the master of your emotions.

Yes, because those attributes display complete control over emotions rather than the other way around.

Exactly. "Seven one six."

How do you activate that?

Your emotional body is all around you. It is a very simple yet powerful technique. Imagine the number 716. See it displayed horizontally, beneath your feet. You can imagine the 716 is large and you are standing atop it. When you breathe, you feel energy immediately. It is a soft yellow. You'll feel energy and tingling beneath your feet.

Breathe it in, and bring this energy up. You will feel as if you are floating and your connection to Earth is slowly lessening. You will feel light and a little spacey: "seven one six." See the beautiful soft-yellow color, and breathe it in. You will feel tingling under your feet.

Yes, it's a little shaky at first, but in the end, it becomes more stable.

You will release a lot of emotions. This number is connected to Archangel Raphael. Archangel Raphael is the angel to call to balance the emotions and emotional body.

You can place the number 716 in a medicine wheel, in a circle, or in an area that you want to shift. Suppose you want to sell a house. Make a medicine wheel on the property, and write the number 716 in the center. Then have the family members stand in the circle on this number, 716. By doing this, the energy will shift. That land can be healed. You will feel a difference, "seven one six."

The Physical Body — 999

The next number, 999 [nine nine nine], is very powerful. This is the earth number in the physical body. The number 9 represents the ability to live as God, to experience your full essence in a physical body. When you add the numbers together [9 + 9 + 9 = 27], you get 27, and when you add 27 [2 + 7 = 9], the result, again, is 9.

Close your eyes and open both palms. Imagine the number 9 on your left palm, the number 9 on your right palm, and another 9 atop your head. Breathe it in. This is a beautiful orange color. Immediately you will feel energy in your hands: nine. Tone this deeply — "nine."

Nine (9). [Repeats several times.]

"Nine." Slowly the number will fade, and you will feel energy in your palms.

I can feel this in my feet too.

Yes, and energy will start spinning. It might make a spiral, and it could take a while. There might be colors above the third eye: "nine."

Okay. What I feel initially from this is a great amount of motivation to do all these practices.

So when you do this exercise, you will anchor Earth's spirit fully into your body because everything, including creation, happens on Earth. Since you hold Earth within you, your creation will manifest much more quickly. It is said that you are Earth.

We carry some of Earth's spirit in us.

Not some, 100 percent. The elements are part of Earth, and you came from Earth's spirit, combining all the elements. It has been said that heaven and Earth exist within you. You are the microcosm and the macrocosm. You need to bring Earth into you. This is one of the reasons many people are not able to manifest things in life. They do spiritual practices, but because they have not activated the earth element within their physical bodies, not much happens.

Structures built on grid lines remain sacred for a long time. Look at the pyramids. Look at the temples of Bali, the temples of Angkor Wat in Cambodia, or St. Paul's Cathedral in London. They are all built on grid lines. They are all still standing. These are very powerful vortexes of energy.

You have grids in your body and on the earth, and you must activate them. When you activate the grid in your body (Earth is in your body) and anchor the energy of your intention in your meditation, you feel good energy and you can anchor into that space. You carry that energy with you.

Often when people meditate, chant, or attend a workshop together, they feel good, but when they go home, they go back to their usual energy.

Yes, they can't sustain it.

Why not? Because they have not anchored into the earth. When you anchor into the earth, the energy will stay there as a grid. There are twelve grids in the body. It will stay there. You must anchor your energy with the earth, and the earth will let you create from that place. It will be a prominent and magnificent creation. Do you see the difference now?

Yes, I do. It's making a lot of sense — earth numbers, nine nine nine [999].

The Galactic Body — 1027

The number for the galactic body is 1027 [one zero two seven]. This galactic number is related to the seven chakras in your body. When you add the numbers [1 + 0 + 2 + 7 = 10], the sum is 10, which is reduced [1 + 0 = 1] to 1.

Once this number is activated, you can tap into galactic consciousness. The number 1027 is like a beautiful sacred geometry pattern. It's as if there is a half-moon on top, and beneath the half-moon, there is a pyramid. One side of the pyramid is missing. The half-moon holds the number 1027.

Visualize this geometric pattern atop your head, and breathe it in. You will slowly see a soft shower of light coming into you, a soft pale white. Allow the energy to just flow through you. It is very subtle. When you do this, you might see devas, deities, gods, and goddesses appear. They watch over you. They are flying over you. How do you feel, brother?

Well, it is very subtle but very fine. I would need some practice to really feel this. But I can sense some of this.

The Solar Body — 1239

We are taking you through the ascension process, and the next number is for the solar level. The solar level is connected to the fifteenth chakra, which is about 5 feet above you. The solar number is 1239 [one two three nine], which totals 15 [1 + 2 + 3 + 9 = 15].

Yes, or 6.

This represents directing to the solar consciousness. You will be able to see the place where many soul imprints are stored.

What are soul imprints?

Soul imprints are memories of past-life experiences that are embedded in the cells. At a much deeper level, there are soul imprints of your experiences in higher-dimensional realities.

In other words, lifetimes not on Earth?

No, it is not a lifetime, not as lifetimes in the higher sense of reality. We are talking about existing in the fifth and up to the twenty-first dimensions, where you never had a physical body. You are a lightbeing, a particle of light. Everything is embedded in this place — solar light.

Visualize solar light as the star of Melchizedek. This looks like the Star of David. Visualize this star around you, and inside it the number 1239 [one two three nine] is displayed horizontally and also vertically. It passes horizontally through your navel and goes vertically from the top of your head to your feet. And this star is big: one two three nine. Just breathe it in.

Is there a color associated with this?

Platinum. This star contracts and expands as you breathe. Most of the time, it is expanding. You become part of this huge star, and there is no more you, only the star and its numbers. That means you have become a nonphysical being. Breathe it in. How do you feel, brother?

Well, it's pretty amazing. I mean, I'm getting inklings of "nonphysicality," if that's a good word.

Exactly. This is what we want you to come to. That means, as you said, there is no more body; you have become an energetic being.

Just beingness.

Exactly, exactly. Just imagine going on for 20 minutes. You would be completely lost — there would be no more you. You would be a sense.

There is no more physicality.

You are just an essence of light, a tiny dot of light. It is incredible, and you are this. You are called the particles of God. You become one with God, a tiny particle with incredible power. See the atom of you. It is white, and in mythology, these are called atma — the divine soul, the solar light.

The Universal Body — 1664

Next is the universal number embedded in human beings. This universal number is related to the sixteenth chakra, which is about 6.5 feet above you. The number is 1664 [one six six four]. The sum of these numbers [1 + 6 + 6 + 4 = 17] is 17, which can be reduced [1 + 7 = 8] to 8.

This is a place of universal creation where everything exists and is then drawn into the void. It merges with the void, goes into a black hole, and is birthed from there. So this is a place of existence and nonexistence. This is a place of inbreath and out-breath, where everything is created and then returns to its original form — pure creative energy. It bursts forth into a supernova, bringing light, and then it slowly returns to the black hole.

There is no death. There is no beginning. There is no end. It is continuous. This is called ebb and flow in a human being, ebb and flow of the God force within you. It is beautiful, brother.

Yes, it is beautiful.

This is the sixteenth chakra, 6.5 feet above the head. It is represented by the infinity symbol.

Which is like a figure 8.

A figure 8, yes, but there are eight figure 8s, all combined and joined and intertwined. They are stacked on top of each other

It's sort of like petals of a flower. Would that be what it looks like?

Yes. Now imagine this symbol in a beautiful platinum color, and breathe it in. In the center of the eights [the eight infinity signs], you have the number 1664.

You will be amazed. The energy will start pouring in front of you, 8 inches in front of your heart. It will flow from the front to the back, opening the high heart center in the back of your body with a beautiful white light. In a matter of minutes, you could be spaced out in another reality. There could be tears, crying. Just breathe it in. If you like, you can chant along with this.

Should I chant the number one six six four?

No. Chant "Om. Om."

Om.

"Om. Om. Om."

This is very familiar to me. I have to say that it feels like Egypt, like a temple in Egypt. I mean, like I've done this before. I don't know whether that makes any sense.

Can you feel the energy?

Yeah, there's a remembrance here of this.

Exactly, the remembrance of the god that you are and a beautiful space.

The Multiuniversal Body — 1991

The next number is for the multiuniverse, which is also part of your reality because you have bodies on Earth, the galactic, the solar, and multiuniversal levels. This is directly related to the thirty-third chakra, which is 10 feet above you. It is also called the Adam chakra. You are a species of Adam, and the number is 1991. This is reduced to 2 [$1 + 9 + 9 + 1 = 20$; $2 + 0 = 2$]. It means, you exist fully present on Earth, *and* you exist fully present in higher realities. You have one foot fully planted in your Earth experience in a physical body and one foot fully planted in universal energy. You live in both worlds.

This is what master Jesus did. He was completely in touch with the power of God and also completely in touch with the average person. He showed that, did he not?

Yeah. It's amazing.

He walked as the master. He was fully aligned with everyday realities — dancing, taking a bath, doing everyday work — and he was always connected with spirit. He always talked about it.

Human beings need to come to the place where they are fully involved in everyday life, never running away from it — experiencing every situation and every moment, enjoying food, taking a shower, going out for a walk — knowing every experience is a blessing, as you are connected to the very spirit that produced all of it. This is a place of absolute mastery.

The number 1991 [one nine nine one] is the thirty-third chakra, which is directly related to Archangel Metatron. He is an incredible master, an archangel who supports humanity with so much love. We encourage all human beings who read this or who will come to know about this to call on this beautiful archangel, for he can guide you and take you through the ascension process.

Is that true for everyone, not just me, personally?

Everyone. Now, how do you contact Archangel Metatron? Think his number, 1991. Imagine a big circle around you and a small circle that extends from you. There is also a third circle that is smaller than and in front of the second circle.

To help me visualize this, are you speaking of two-dimensional circles or three-dimensional spheres?

Imagine a cone, okay? At the opening — the base — there is a big circle; at the middle, there is a smaller circle; and near the end, there is the smallest circle. Just breathe it in. It is a beautiful platinum color, and inside the cone, you see the sacred geometry of a tetrahedron and an octahedron. Just breathe it in.

The circles will start spinning. They will go above you, below you, or through you, like particles — atoms and molecules — flying all over. It looks like the electricity symbol, like an atom with many electrons circling a nucleus, and it has many lines crisscrossing each other that create a flame of energy. Just breathe it in. Make the sound "arum."

Arum.

"Arum."

Arum [repeats several times].

The flame will not consume you. You will be in the flame of Archangel Metatron. "Arum."

What I feel is a sense of being in some sort of interdimensional fire. It's very purifying. It's certainly not hot.

No, this is the fire of Archangel Metatron.

Yes, like an energy field.

Exactly. You're joining with the force of the multiuniversal energy. Metatron is taking you to join with that part of you.

The Omni-Universal Body — 2799

The next one is called the omni-universe. You exist in the omni-universe as part of the energy of the Great Central Sun, an energy of the Creator. You are a speck of light in the overall energy of the Creator, and this is connected to the forty-second chakra. It is about 4.5 meters above your head. The number is 2799 [two seven nine nine].

The symbol for the omni-universe is the ankh. Visualize a very large ankh. It extends to about 4.5 meters above your head. It goes through your entire body and then down very deep into the ground. The ankh is gold, and 2799 is displayed on it vertically.

It's amazing. I mean, I can feel this. The feeling is confidence.

Close your eyes. Just imagine this golden ankh inside of you with its number (2799), and you are in the middle of this golden color. Its gold is around you and goes through you. Now make the sound "narom."

Narom.

Be careful because you will ignite incredible energy. As the number 2799 [two seven nine nine] starts spinning, you will feel energy hitting your third eye area. And the number will spin very fast.

Visualize this number in your own way. "Narom. Narom."

It was like being welcomed into a higher space. There was a sense of being welcomed.

"Narom" means "coming home."

This is very powerful; there is a feeling of great benevolence.

You will feel a lot of expansion; your body is expanding. You have become very tall. Narom. You will see that your body is still human, but it has a different reality to it, and you have become quite a huge figure.

It feels as if my body has become less dense. It's more etheric, like I could walk through a wall.

Exactly. "Narom."

Well, I feel really good.

•   •   •

This is the Family of God. We want to thank the people who support us, Master Mahareya, Guru Rinpoche, King Akhenaton, celestial beings of light, Master Kuthumi, and all other angels and guardians who are with us today. More than 15,000 energies are watching this transmission right now.

Well, I feel special.

We say thank you, thank you, thank you. Until we meet again.

Release Fear

Family of God, Osiris, Akhenaton, and Isis

Family of God: Hello. We would like to include the energies of the Celestial Beings of Light combined with our energies in this session. Isis is considered the mother of all lineages and all orders. This includes the Order of the Rose, the Order of the Golden Dawn, the Order of the Magdalenes, and other orders as well. Everything came from Isis. Now we will discuss ascension key 28 — releasing fear using the Osiris code.

Beloved Osiris is called the god of resurrection. What does resurrection mean? Resurrection simply means a new beginning, a new way of life, discarding the old. This is stepping into a new body of light. True initiation takes place with Osiris, and connecting with Osiris can help you overcome the fear of death. Initiations in Egyptian temples were ventures into the underworld, where Osiris judged the initiate. This is an archetypal story. Connecting with Osiris can help you overcome your fear of death.

Once you activate these codes, you are ready to step into the halls of initiation. When you feel comfortable with them, particularly the code of Yeshua, this could be very powerful. Some people will take a couple of days or weeks to anchor the energy of this initiation fully into their beings because it could shake up their whole bodies. When it is fully integrated, it is likely that your energy will increase, and it will help you to set a new course.

The fear of death happens because there is fear of the unknown. "What is going to happen to me afterward?" Many people carry deep shame and regret before they die, and feeling judged, they do not know what is going to happen. Much of this comes from religions, and because they are unable to see what will happen, they distrust it. The root of any fear is the feeling of powerlessness. When you think that a situation is not in your control, you feel fearful.

First, you need to define the exact situations that make you feel powerless and fearful. How does fear start? Fear is a negative state of being. It arises when you lose faith and when you forget to surrender. When you do not surrender, you resist. There can be no fear in true faith and surrender.

This goes counter to how human beings are programmed to stay alive. Is that not true?

Yes, of course. The essence of surrender is that you let go of expectations. You could say, "Because I am dying at this time, I will let go of what I expect on the other side." Let go of your ideas about how your life should go, and totally give yourself up to divine guidance, accepting what is happening at that moment. The moment you surrender and let go, you are free of fear. You realize that what was happening has a divine reason, for nothing is random, including death. This is important to remember. So much fear is created when your logical mind tries to plan your future or to understand what is happening at a given moment. Major causes of fear are repetitive negative thoughts and preconceived ideas or judgments about a situation.

When you have fear, you create blocks in your spinal column — blocks to the movement of energy through the spinal column, which is where your quantum self energy exists. The larger part of you exists in your spinal column. When you carry fear, this energy is blocked and unable to move. When this energy stops moving, you feel disconnected from your quantum self and very alone. You feel like you are a nobody. You are just one single human being. You are unable to connect with the larger aspects of yourself. Fear and insecurity stop the flow of kundalini energy.

Release Fear from Past Lifetimes

So much fear is carried from past lifetimes. It is carried in your blood. Ask that all the fear codes of death you have brought from other lifetimes be released. Fear caught in your blood from this lifetime or other lifetimes stops cosmic energy from being released. There are angels to help you with this — the white angels of light. Their principle work is to support humanity to release all fear brought from this lifetime and other lifetimes, particularly the fear of death. Release the fear into the ethers, and ask the white angels to process it for you. This is very important.

When you come to the Chamber of Initiation with Osiris, what he is really examining in you is not whether your heart is pure, as the story says, or whether it is lighter than a feather. He only looks at whether you have fear. When there is fear, your heart is heavy. This is not natural, so you feel cut off from your essence. As you enter the Chamber of Initiation, if you are able to hold your essence, refocus all the energy in your spinal column, and breathe into it. This way, you will be able to connect with your essence. Close your eyes and focus on your spinal column. Breathe into your spinal column slowly, hold your breath, slowly take it up through your crown, and then release it above your head.

I feel fear in my solar plexus, which is on the other side of my body.

Wherever it is, fear is not only in one chakra. It is in almost all the chakras, but when you start breathing and releasing the fear in the spinal column, much of the fear in the chakras can also be released. When you are fearful, you become immobilized. It stops you in your tracks. Your power is stopped, and you become like an animal. Animals can sense your fear. If you're fearful, they will attack you.

People will take advantage of others when they feel fear. The initiation with Osiris is simply about your willingness to surrender to the experience you are having in the moment and to get in touch with your pure essence. If you are willing, then you can ask for the initiation of the white feather with Osiris. What will he do? He will touch your heart with his white feather, which has a golden tip.

The Initiation of Osiris
in the Temple of Resurrection

Close your eyes now to experience this. Call forward Osiris to speak for an initiation.

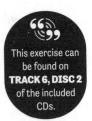

This exercise can be found on **TRACK 6, DISC 2** of the included CDs.

I call forward Osiris at this time.

Osiris: Hello, my brother. I am with my beloved Isis. Welcome to the new you, and what a grand time to do this in the month of August, when there is so much powerful energy and influence. Let me ask you what I ask everybody: Why have you come here? You have given the answer before, but I would like to hear it. I will remind you of the answer: "I have come here to rejoin the god that I am."

Yes.

Is this your answer?

Yes.

Gently close your eyes. Now I take the white feather with the golden tip in my hands, and I touch your heart. I gently touch it three times from the top to the bottom. There is an opening in your heart. I place the feather in your heart. Imagine a beautiful white feather with a golden tip in your heart, and breathe. Do you feel a lightness come into your heart? This is an extension of the feather. You might see geometric patterns, shapes, and colors, including stars. Breathe into these.

I will ask you some questions now. Are you ready to serve the truth?

My answer is yes.

Are you ready to embrace the love that is in you?

Yes.

Are you ready to serve humanity from now onward?

Yes.

Through your body, through your mind, and through your soul in its full integrity and truth on all levels, are you ready to serve? Is this your highest truth?

This is my highest truth, and this is my intention. I cannot guarantee that I am ready, but I certainly intend to be there while doing these things.

Let it be recorded in the book of records what you said today. Let this be part of your akash. I place my hands behind your neck, activating several powerful frequencies of light. See a beautiful golden pyramid appear and touch the base of your neck.

Breathe into the golden pyramid, and energy will come from the top of the pyramid and enter the base of your neck, flowing into your body. Breathe several times. Anchor the golden pyramid within you eternally.

I anchor this golden pyramid within me eternally.

"For I am the carrier of the golden pyramid energy within me."

For I am the carrier of the golden pyramid energy within me.

"I will always protect this golden pyramid energy within me. I will sanctify it. I will honor it because it is sacred energy within me."

I will protect, honor, and sanctify this golden pyramid energy within me.

Just breathe it in. Open your palms, and now I place a necklace in your hands made of beautiful amethyst crystals, shining brilliantly. I ask you to place this necklace around your neck. Feel its vibration fill you with its incredible amethyst light.

Yes, I can feel this.

Your entire being feels it. Absorb this energy.

Family of God: Now the great King Akhenaton steps forward. He touches your forehead, and he asks you initiation questions.

Akhenaton: Are you ready to hold the law — the law of one — as your truth from now onward?

I am ready.

Will you align only with this law or to everything else?

Only the law of one.

Simply say: "This is my truth from now on. I am fully aligned with the law."

This is my truth from now on, for I am fully aligned with the law of one.

Osiris: Breathe it in. Now is your greatest test. Sister Isis steps forward and asks you a very important question.

Isis: Are you ready to join with your twin flame?

Yes. I would do anything for that.

Your twin flame is magnificent, a larger part, the I Am part of you.

I ask you to say, "I allow the energy of my twin flame." See a pouring of light from way above you come into you like a waterfall of white light.

I allow the energy of the twin flame to come within me.

"I accept the love and the energy of the twin flame within me now."

I accept the energy of the twin flame within me now.

"I embrace my twin flame."

I embrace my twin flame.

"I become one with it."

I become one with it.

Osiris: Well, brother, we took you through an initiation process today. This initiation is only given when asked with the purest love and intention to join the highest parts of you. It must be done in reverence, with sacredness, and with a sincere heart, seeking the reunion of yourself.

This is very powerful. I am so lifted now. I have worked with Isis before, but I have no conscious exposure to Osiris, and he feels so familiar. It is opening something so special within me.

Every day, work with the golden pyramid at the base of your neck and then with the necklace you are wearing. You will feel the sacred energy well up within you from now on. This is Osiris with Isis and King Akhenaton.

Thank you. Thank you so much.

Family of God: Hello, dear brother. We took you through this process today so that you could experience and share this energy. This energy will stay with you, and you can connect with it anytime you want. Remember this moment in time, for it will be recorded in your history. Every time human beings are ready to accept the larger part of themselves, it is recorded. This is a special moment in the history of this planet.

I feel really honored to be given this.

The Three Resurrection Codes of Osiris
Code One

Here is a sound to support the first resurrection code: "ma sa re." As you make this sound, cup your left hand in front of your sternum. The fingers of your right hand are splayed, and your right thumb presses into the

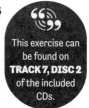

This exercise can be found on **TRACK 7, DISC 2** *of the included CDs.*

palm of your cupped left hand [see figure 28.1]. Close your eyes, and make the sound "ma sa re."

Ma sa re.

Very good. A few times more and you will feel flames in your third eye and in your body. Say this nine times: "ma sa re."

Ma sa re [chants nine times]. It is totally activating my sixth chakra, my third eye. It seems like a portal into other dimensions. The chakra is on fire, and it is opening into other dimensions.

Code Two

Cup your left hand. Your right thumb and pinky finger touch each other, and the other fingers are splayed. The right thumb and pinky finger touch the palm of the cupped left hand, and this is held in front of the navel [see figure 28.2]. Make the sound "ye hu de me." When you do this, you will feel the energy ground you into a new frequency. You will go deeper and deeper, and it will manifest energy in your legs. Do this nine times.

It seems important to have your feet flat on the ground.

Yes, you will feel intense energy grounding you there.

Ye hu de me [chants nine times]. I can feel this. It feels like being, what you said, an original human, and it's making me feel very at home on Earth.

Because you live on Earth in a earth body, all your energy must be anchored into the earth so that it can rise into your physical life. You can use this higher energy because it is anchored into the ground, and it becomes available to you to use for creating higher realities in your life.

This is very beautiful. This is part of the Osiris and Isis initiation. It is like grounding and finishing the initiation. Is that correct?

Yes.

Code Three

Osiris: Hold your hands in the prayer position so that your wrists are in front of your forehead [see figure 28.3], and make the sound "om harr." Hold your hands in the prayer position in front of your heart [see figure 28.4], and make the sound "sum harr." Place your hands beneath your navel in the prayer position, and make the sound "ru maar." Place your hands by your knees in the prayer position pointing downward [see figure 28.5], and make the sound "bra hoor." Extend both arms out

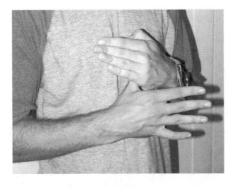

Figure 28.1   Figure 28.2

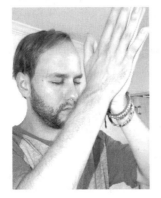
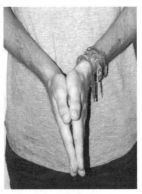
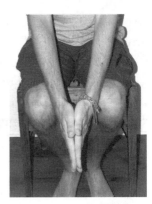

Figure 28.3   Figure 28.4   Figure 28.5

Figures 28.1–28.5. Mudras to activate the resurrection codes of Osiris

to your sides so that your body forms a T with your palms facing down, and make the sound "moooong."

These steps will integrate the energies of the activation throughout your being. You might feel energy in your palms and fingers.

I feel those feelings.

Say, "It remains. I have come back home. I am joined with Earth once again in service to humanity."

It remains. I have come back home. I am joined with Earth once again in service to humanity.

We bless you, and all others who are on the path of seeking God within them. May your crown be open. Let the light and flowers of light pour into you. Imagine your crown is open and a shower of light is falling with white petals pouring into your head.

Thank you.

Family of God: Through this code, you are able to access the highest frequency. Do this for 1 month, and practice this Osiris initiation daily. After your resurrection, he will guide you.

Osiris carries the energy of Archangel Michael, the forebear of new consciousness. There are three codes. The first code is an accurate rendition of the code of Osiris. It goes up and then down your spinal cord from the crown down to the hips. The second code goes from the crown down the spinal column to your legs and then to your feet.

This is the kundalini, so the second code is the kundalini.

Yes.

I feel this total vertical integration from the feet all the way up to the crown. The third code I don't really understand. Part of me wants to cry. I don't know what is going on here.

This is called the law of integration.

So this third code opens service to humanity. Is that correct?

Yes, service to humanity. It comes from humility and deep love for humanity. It is called the mother energy. This is the code of Isis. When you grow exponentially, you are much more compassionate to everything and everyone, and you can interject mother energy. Mother always holds and embraces everyone. We are the Family of God with the celestial beings.

Could you explain who the celestial beings are?

Human beings are celestial, but the celestial beings are one of the supporting energies under the direction of the Council of Creators to support humanity, assisting ascension. We believe that the information in this book will serve humanity for a long time.

I am honored. Thank you.

Ínitiate Kundalini Movement

The Family of God

Family of God: Hello, brother of love. We are the Family of God. Enjoy the precious moments. Be good to your family. As human beings grow, they express their experiences of God. So enjoy every moment with your beautiful family. Thank you for participating in this joint adventure.

Now we will discuss ascension key 29 — initiating kundalini. We have a very interesting guest, the energy of the snake and ascension. You might ask, "Why are snakes so important for ascension?" The awakening of the kundalini is likened to the movement of a snake in the spinal column. The energy moves like waves. But there is much more than that.

Why are people afraid of snakes? This fear was manipulated, just as your DNA was manipulated. The kundalini takes the shape of a coiled snake within a human being. Snakes are wonderful creatures and should not be feared. Some have poison, but they only use their poison for self-defense. Human minds are poisoned with fear. Like snakes, when humans are provoked or attacked, they use the poison (in their minds) to harm others (through words or physical action).

Snakes have a very important role. They can teach many things. They are always in touch with Mother Earth because they carry the Earth spirit. They crawl on the ground. They crawl on rocks. They crawl in trees. They swim in water. Not many creatures have the capacity to be in all these places. What do they say? Snakes say, "I am connected to the elements, the spirit of Earth, of which I was created, so that I can teach human beings how they must never forget their roots — what they are made of, the elements."

The great king cobra has a physical hood and an etheric V-shaped pattern between its eyes. This is a place of connection to all that heals. You have the same etheric pattern on your forehead. Through this opening, you can connect with all that heals and experience All That Is. The king cobra never forgets his existence and the force through which he was created.

Some snakes carry jewels on their heads — etheric diamonds of light. Human beings also carry etheric diamonds in the middle of their brains, emitting a soft-purple light. Both have similar energies.

In the Egyptian tradition, there are many paintings and images of snakes. Every temple has pictures of snakes. The Egyptians understood the significance of the energy of snakes, which are completely in harmony and in balance with the elements. They also carry an incredible light on the top of their heads.

People who have taken the hallucinogenic drug ayahuasca often see visions of snakes. In Indian mythology, the great god Vishnu sits on a coiled serpent, and the hood of the serpent protects him. When Master Buddha meditated, a big king cobra opened its hood over him to protect him from the rain. The Maya also knew about the significance of the snake, and they made drawings of snakes.

Get the Kundalini Moving

You can connect with the great snake being. The being you can call is named Nag De Va, Utior. "Nag De Va" means the goddess of snakes, but this deity is not shaped like a snake. She is rather round and emanates a beautiful soft-blue light. You can ask her to anchor her light in your base chakra to move your kundalini. This blue light is like a lantern that leads the kundalini, moving it up the back of your body all the way to your crown chakra. This is a gift given to human beings from the benevolent Arcturians.

Now, my brother, bring your attention to your base chakra, and say, "I call on Nag De Va."

I call on Nag De Va.

See a beautiful blue sphere of light settle into your base chakra. Focus there, and breathe. You will see this blue light slowly move up. Attached to the blue light is your kundalini energy. It looks like a snake, and the blue light gently moves up, followed by the kundalini.

Make the sound "ra ha seka emmai. Ra ha seka emmai. Ra ha seka emmai." Let the blue light go up into your crown. Behind the blue light is a beautiful snake. Now it spreads its hood over your crown and your brain. "Ra ha seka emmai. Ra ha seka emmai. Ra ha seka emmai."

Now open your palms and say, "I bring this kundalini shakti into my hands."

I bring this kundalini shakti into my hands.

Do you see the blue light coming into your palms?

Yes, I can feel this. This is quite amazing.

"Ra ha seka emmai. Ra ha seka emmai. Ra ha seka emmai." When the blue light comes for people who have worked on their spiritual journeys for a long time, the kundalini will follow the blue light very gently. But if there are blocks, the kundalini will have a hard time. It is as if a wall has been built. Pushing through that wall can some-times be difficult. But after doing this simple exercise, you will see the kundalini move or gently flow to the crown. It's very simple, brother.

Put your full attention on the sound, brother: "Ra ha seka emmai. Ra ha seka emmai. Ra ha seka emmai. Ra ha seka emmai. Ra ha seka emmai. Ra ha seka emmai. Ra ha seka emmai." For this exercise to have the natural benefit, it must be done daily for 45 days. The kundalini will rise gently with no discomfort to the physical body: "Ra ha seka emmai. Ra ha seka emmai. Ra ha seka emmai."

* * *

I have one question. You mentioned that in human beings, there was an etheric diamond in the middle of the brain emitting light. Is that the pineal gland?

No. The pineal gland is inside the medulla oblongata in the back of the head, exactly behind the third eye. In the middle of the brain, there are two hemispheres. It is between the two hemispheres. There is important DNA there.

Inspire Creative Action and Self-Confidence

Thunder and Lightning and the Family of God

Thunder and Lightning: Hello, my friends. I walk in partnership with my beloved brother. I am known as Indra, and my partner is Mitra. We hold certain frequencies of light and energy. We now discuss ascension key 30 — creative action and self-confidence.

The Creator has placed many beings on this planet, in this universe, and in this galaxy to perform various tasks. For example, there is a spirit for the rain and a spirit for the clouds. All perform their own tasks. They work in balance and move forward in harmony, supporting humanity's evolution.

We are also here to support humanity's evolution. The role assigned to us is to create electrical energy to generate new thought patterns, designs, structures of land, or specific inventions. Our work is to produce thunder and lightning, but we do this in collaboration and harmony with Mother Earth, Father Sky, the spirit of the Moon, the spirit of the Sun, and the spirit of ocean waves.

Waves communicate to Mother Earth. They act as a feedback system, informing her about particular areas on the planet at certain times. Mother Earth will coordinate with the mountains, the wind, and your soul. Many things go into the physical phenomena you observe. You might say that it is just raining, but there was preparation before the rains arrived.

Mother Earth tries to bring the best of everything; however, there are beings who do not want Mother Earth to help people. They do not want beneficial energies because they want to keep people in darkness. Mother Earth can bring rain to the planet in a matter of minutes, but there are many factors there. There is karmic energy. There is the aspect of learning life lessons. Thunder and lightning bring new thought patterns of energy to be dispersed throughout the land.

An example is the Hollywood filmmaker George Lucas. His movies are entertaining and informative. They have opened the imagination of many people about other life forms. Television programs such as *Star Trek* have done the same. How do these creative people draw their energy and inspiration? How did George Lucas come up with beautiful and imaginative scenarios? He had to first conceive the ideas. They were given by dragon spirits after obtaining permission. The inspiration was downloaded into Earth. Certain people are receptive to these ideas and can work with them.

Another such person is Steven Spielberg. He believed in certain ideas. He did not have doubt. The same could be said of Albert Einstein. Some people come here to support humanity. They are wired a little differently. They have specific goals. Many people have several life purposes. But some people have only one life purpose, which is to create something special that will benefit larger communities of people. The dragons, along with us, send out information, wisdom, and guidance for humanity. This has increased since the shift of 2012.

Weather patterns have shifted during the past ten years. The weather is getting hotter in some places. Winter is longer in other places, and there have been times of heavy rain in some places. The climate is changing. When the weather is wet, people are more open and receptive. When people live in dry areas, they are not as open. The purpose of rain is communicated through the clouds. The clouds communicate with Mother Earth and the wind. They say how the rain should be — just a drizzle or a heavy downpour. It is all coordinated.

When the weather is wet, people are in a much more receptive state. They are more in touch with their essences. It is not that they are completely awakened, but there is a higher probability they will be in tune with their inner essence during times of rain. A lot of creativity can happen with rain. Look at your area, the Berkshires of western Massachusetts. Many writers have lived there. They found the area to be beautiful, and it is still very popular. Nature supported them. Their creativity was supported. Norman Rockwell went to that area and created paintings there.

Activate Inspiration, Self-Confidence, and Creativity through Indra

We, the consciousness of thunder and lightning, disseminate the energy of inspiration. This is done through rains, thunder, and lightning. There are places in your body that connect to our energy. Look at your fingers. Each finger has three parts with two joints. The backs of your fingers are directly connected to us. You feel this more when you touch your wrist. These places contain energy and mini chakras. Once these are activated, you will feel the energy of fire.

Bring your attention to the back of the middle finger of your right hand. Touch the knuckle with the index finger of your left hand. Inhale, and visualize a yellow-orange vortex. Make the sound "inmi."

Inmi.

Now spread the fingers of both hands, focus on the bones, and say, "Inmi."

Inmi. Inmi. Inmi. It is starting to tingle.

When you activate this, you will take creative actions, and you will begin to believe in yourself.

So this activates creativity and self-confidence. Is that correct?

Yes. It helps you believe in yourself, and then you can take creative action. Along with this come faith and trust in your abilities.

When you close your eyes, you can feel an energy come from your hands. This is seen as fire. It goes through your third eye, and you will see flames. You will definitely feel energy moving there. Make the sound "inmi" a few more times.

Inmi. Inmi. Inmi.

You could even feel energy flowing from your hands into your arms.

I do. I feel that particularly in my forearms.

So we support bringing new and inspired ideas and taking action. This will stay activated always.

My hands feel different. It's as if there is some substance that wasn't there before.

As you know, this has never been done before. Now it has been activated.

So someone on the path of ascension can do this to become inspired for creative purposes.

Yes, to have faith that inspiration will come to them. For ascension, you must learn to have faith in yourself, in your ability to master life, and then you can move forward.

That is very beautiful and very uplifting.

Connect with the Stars, Planets, and Galaxies

Now we ask you to bring your attention to the space between the inside of your lips and your teeth. Focus on this place.

Breathe in the energy of Indra into this place. Breathe it in through your nose, and focus the energy on that area. You might start feeling energy going into your brain, your third eye, and the space above that.

I do. I feel it immediately.

Can you do this nine times?

I have now done that nine times, and my impression is that it affects speech.

It totally affects your brain, once you fully activate this area. Exhale, and bring this energy beneath your hairline.

It is amazing. I feel that it connects me to something much higher than myself.

It connects you to the reality of the stars, the planets, and the galaxies. Just imagine doing this for 5 minutes. You will become one with them. Your consciousness will expand.

It's amazing. I don't know what it is, but it's clearly not me.

We are bringing techniques that can expand consciousness. The more you expand your consciousness, the closer you become to your calling or your goal. Your goal is ascension. When you are able to connect with the stars and the galaxies, you are in a very high state of energy. Then you will be able to bring that energy into your body and make it a part of your reality. You will be in a very high state. When you are in this place, you will feel inspired and guided. And I, Indra, stay in your fingers. Mitra stays where you brought the energy near your hairline.

This is amazing. I have a somewhat mental question. Would you call yourself a deva, a spirit, a master, or a God? This is for the readers.

We would say that we are devas. Devas support humanity in humility. We have been assigned the role to communicate these secret teachings to people at this time. So we are now able to bring this information forward.

Presumably, during Earth's history some people have practiced this. Is that correct, or has this been done in secret?

Of course. There are many secret teachings. Some are from the ancient land of Ireland. There are also secret teachings in the lands of Israel, Egypt, India, Greece, Mongolia, and Russia. There are many secret teachings. We believe that it is time to bring these out so that they are not exclusively used in secret. This is for people in general. We are now in a new world. People want to have experiences right away; otherwise, they will lose faith or not believe.

Or they will not be interested.

Exactly. Times are changing. We also work with and inspire the snake kingdom. During rainy times, snakes come out of the ground. They enjoy the rain and the thunder. The peacocks also enjoy thunder and lightning. They open their tails and dance. These animals represent the qualities of ascension, the ability to dance as masters. The peacock dances the dance of freedom.

The snake represents the ability to stay connected to the ground. Even when you go very high in consciousness, a snake is still connected to the ground. When a snake climbs up trees, it is still connected to the ground. It can crawl on rocks, and it can swim in water, but it always stays connected. Wherever it goes, it never loses touch with its original connection. It will still live in humility and be humble. It will be connected to the very element that produced it, which is Mother Earth. To a human being, this means: "No matter how far I go, I will always be humble and connected to the first spirit."

This is the end of the discourse for today. We believe this has the potential to shift the realities of many people.

I believe that too. It is very good.

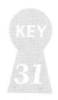

Attune the Body's Internal Compass

The Family of God, Archangel Gabriel, Mohamed,
Master Yeshua, Archangel Michael, and the Shepherd Boy

*Note: These practices were channeled in Israel during a journey to the
Holy Land undertaken by Rae, Robert, and thirty-five fellow travelers
in July 2017. The Family of God asked for this to be included.*

The Family of God: The Dome of the Rock is a seventh-century
mosque built on the site of the Second Temple on the Temple
Mount in Jerusalem. Many people believe that the dome shelters
a rock that is the energetic navel of Earth. Light is beamed to this
rock, and from there, it is distributed to other sacred sites on the
planet and from those sites to human beings. This discussion is
about ascension key 31 — attuning the body's inner compass. The
following practice will reset your internal compass to align with
Earth's navel.

   Archangel Gabriel and Mohamed: Everything in the universe
has sound frequencies. You can program your ears to attune to the
frequencies of the stone at the Dome of the Rock. When you open
yourself to sound frequencies (received behind your ears), you will

understand how to work with your internal compass and attune to the frequencies of this rock.

Close your eyes, focus on your ears, and tone the sound "sa la ma ha." You will immediately feel energy behind your ears. When you make this sound, you reset the sound frequencies of your compass. You are directing the energy of this sound frequency to be in alignment with your compass. Do this for 13 to 21 days, and you will always hear the celestial voice of your soul.

You can augment what you hear with your internal compass by wearing an earring in your right ear. Diamond earrings are the most effective.

Activate the Shepherd's DNA Code

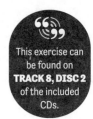

This exercise can be found on **TRACK 8, DISC 2** of the included CDs.

Master Yeshua, Archangel Michael, and the Shepherd Boy: This is called the shepherd's code. A shepherd leads his flock to safety. Through the shepherd's code, your DNA will lead you to your truth.

1. Close your eyes, raise your hands in prayer position, and make the sound "hum, hum, hum."
2. Open the fingers of your right hand. The Shepherd Boy is going to give you his stick. Feel the vibration of the stick in your hand. Breathe it in, and it will start vibrating. Breathe.
3. This stick goes into the back of your body. It aligns and merges with your spinal column. As you breathe, feel this stick vibrating. It contains the energy of the shepherd who leads people to truth. Feel it vibrating at the back of your body, activating your DNA, clearing your spinal column, and balancing your past, present, and future energies. Be in this space completely.
4. This stick also anchors the energy of Arcturus in you. Your DNA is activating.
5. Stay in this space in silence as these sounds are toned for you: "whoh, whoh, whoh, whoh, wuuu, wuuu, wuma, wuma, wuma, ahhh, ooo, ae, mei, ie, oooo, oooo, ooooo, oooo, oooo, oooo, oooo, ooooo, oooo, oooo, aima, ohayma, oooo, oooo, oooo, ohayma, ohayma, ohayma, ooo, oooo, oooo, ohayma, ohayma, oooo, oooo."
6. Visualize a golden *S* in your medulla oblongata at the base of the back of your neck. This is the DNA of the shepherd's code. It means

you are encompassed in a knowingness that leads you to the highest truth within you. Feel this *S* symbol at the back of your neck.

7. Master Yeshua asks you to open both your hands, palms up, to receive. He places a small lamb in your hands. Hold it. Take it to your heart. Embrace it, and make this statement, "I am leading my sheep to my Father's kingdom. Together, the Father and I are One. I will maintain and remember this connection. I will strengthen this connection from this moment onward. I love my Father more than my life. The Father and I are One."

8. This is the meaning of Jesus holding the sheep. Feel the energy. Don't open your eyes. Stay in this space for a while.

This completes the initiation of the shepherd's code.

Integrate the Universal Body Template

The Family of God

Family of God: Lord Melchizedek is the master of this universe. He holds the frequency for the Earth plane, this galaxy, and billions of planets. Lord Melchizedek is important for ascension because he holds the template for the universal body. When people ascend, there is a shift of the frequency in their physical bodies, and many energetic bodies begin to join their physical bodies. Bodies from other dimensions start to merge.

Here we discuss ascension key 32 — the universal body template. There are many levels of ascension. It takes much time to fully integrate the light, and every person does it differently. The Earth being's ascension integrates the universal body template so that you can exist as a universal being. When that happens, your understanding and experience comes from a universal perspective. The wisdom and light you emit are universal. This is important because the universe contains many realities and many dimensions. When you connect with this energy, you experience aspects of yourself from many dimensions, and you realize that you are bigger than the universe. With that realization and experience, you will not identify with anything. You are bigger than the identity itself.

Many people feel that they are "this," or they are "that," and they rarely define the spiritual revolution that they have undergone. They could say, "I belong to this planet. I identify with that spiritual tradition." Do not identify with anything. Be universal. This is a place of formlessness. "I am the ever-changing formless part of myself." This can only be experienced fully when you embrace and integrate the universal body template, and Lord Melchizedek is the master who initiates people into this body.

Call on Lord Melchizedek to download the universal body template to entirely assimilate this energy in you. You will be able to anchor it fully within you and around you, and into Earth's template, the sky's template, your elemental bodies (earth, air, fire, and water), and the connections you have with the trees, the forests, and the rivers. Part of your energy will go into these bodies. They will hold their energy for you so that you can experience their energies whenever you want, because you will have become part of everything. Lord Melchizedek does this on an individual basis, and it is done by asking that the universal body template be downloaded into you.

The universal body template is downloaded into the seventeen pyramidal structures that exist within you. These pyramids are containers used to store energy. For example, the King's Chamber of the Great Pyramid is a place where energy is held, and you can experience energies when you go there, when you are ready. Call on Lord Melchizedek.

You have the Lord Melchizedek code (and a Metatron code) in your pineal gland. Your pineal gland is much more than you think it is.

The Melchizedek Code Activation

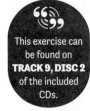

This exercise can be found on **TRACK 9, DISC 2** of the included CDs.

1. Close your eyes, and bring your attention to your medulla oblongata.
2. Ask Lord Melchizedek to download the universal body template into your consciousness.
3. Imagine a thin stream of light coming from your pineal gland. A silver color flows into your neck where it splits into two parts, like a river runs through two tributaries. Both streams flow around your spinal column and enter its base.

4. A beautiful silver light appears in your spinal column. Breathe, and visualize this silver light going all the way up to your twelfth chakra. Don't stop at your head.

5. Breathe again, and see it go all the way down to the earth-star chakra beneath your feet.

6. Bring the light up to your hips, breathe, and visualize it go through your spinal column and all the way up to the twelfth chakra again.

7. Hold it there, and see it come back down, taking it all the way through to your soul-star chakra. This is the energy of the universal body template of Melchizedek running through your spinal column, all the way up and all the way down.

8. You will see an opening in front of your heart. This is a portal to other dimensions. Take the silver light all the way up and all the way down, bring it back up, and send it out in front of your sternum.

9. Breathe it in again. See it go all the way up and then all the way down. Then watch it flow back up, and push it out the front of the sternum. One more time, breathe. See it go up, down, up, and out through this portal.

10. See a silver lotus in front of your heart. See it grow larger and larger. This is the code of Melchizedek. This means you have embraced the universal consciousness of Lord Melchizedek.

11. You will feel warmth in your body and perhaps a bit spaced out initially, but you will hold higher frequencies of light without even identifying that it is part of the universal body.

12. Say, "I am the formless part of myself." See this beautiful lotus of silver light singing in harmony with the breeze.

13. When you keep this portal open, it will emit light. This light will go everywhere in your aura and into other realities. Every part of you in every other reality will feel the vibration of this beautiful lotus.

14. When you wake in the morning or meditate, ask that this lotus be fully awakened so that it becomes part of you. You'll experience greatly expanded consciousness when this happens.

When you are serious in your spiritual practice and this lotus opens, your heart will fully open, and you will experience great compassion and a feeling of love for humanity. Tears of joy will come naturally. When you see an act of kindness or beauty, tears will come because you are experiencing Divine love.

When this lotus opens as you write or channel, masters will introduce you to other realities. You will gain strength, and you will be able to bring forth understanding through channeling or automatic writing.

How do you feel, brother?

I could feel some of what was happening, and I felt a sense of formlessness that I have never experienced before. I could feel that everything was silver. I followed most of what you said with this incredible experience, but obviously I need a lot of practice with this. Something changed.

This is a very profound initiation meditation. You can connect with Lord Melchizedek, the master of this universe. You will experience his grandness through your eyes, your mind, and your heart.

We are with you throughout this journey with the intention to bring understanding. Everyone has the potential to realize and accept who they are — formless beings. We are the Family of God. Thank you and blessings.

Continue the Ascension Journey

The Family of God, Archangel Metatron, Creator, Commander Ashtar, King Akhenaton, Maha Avatar Babaji, and Gaia

Family of God: We are the Family of God. We send light and love to you, your beloved cats, your house, your environment, and to the people of your beautiful country.

Every day when you wake up in the morning, we ask you to extend your arms and visualize beautiful America. Breathe light, and fill this country with light from your heart so that there will be more agreement among people. People will talk to each other without hatred. Hold this space every day for a few minutes, sending light to the country. Your country is a leader. It can show a new vibration to other parts of the world, so always hold your country in light despite what has happened. Hold light for the people.

I will.

This will increase your light inside as well.

Thank you. This country needs all the help it can get right now.

Today, we are accompanied by Archangels Metatron and Gabriel to talk about ascension key 33 — the journey of ascension.

The Ra Mu Ma Code of Ascension

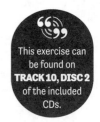

Metatron: Blessed family of light, this is Archangel Metatron. I have been invited to speak today to bring further understanding of the process you call ascension. This word has been used many times, but people do not really understand its meaning. Ascension is not a destination. It is a journey. You are ascending every moment when you take a positive step to increase the light within you. It is the same as liberation. Liberation happens moment by moment as you take positive action to create and integrate more light.

Ascension is a step-based process. When you wake in the morning, ask, "How can I ascend today from the chains I have made for myself — from an old belief system or a thought pattern?" We highly recommend continually seeking to ascend by integrating more light. When you are on the journey doing the exercises that have been given here to the best of your ability, you will surely reach your destination, which is to become light itself.

Today, we wish to talk about an aspect of Arcturus. This is an important aspect in the journey of ascension. The planet Arcturus is a place of gathering. Beings gather there much as a shepherd gathers his sheep in the evening. This is like bringing people back Home. People gather on Arcturus, where they are shown the gateway to move toward ascension. Arcturus is the midway point between All That Is and you. After the Earth plane, you will go to Arcturus for further energy processing and to heal and purify. Then you will be ready to merge with the light.

In Arcturus, there are temples dedicated to this process. The template of your fifth-dimensional consciousness is integrated into you. Make it a point to go to the Temple of Ra Mu Ma on Arcturus daily to join with your fifth-dimensional consciousness. This can raise your frequency considerably. You will be able to bring this higher frequency into the Earth plane in your physical body to solve problems in your life and to heal.

There are many masters on Arcturus — musical masters, energy healing masters, and meditation masters. Meditation masters maintain the equilibrium of the planet by regulating the atmosphere and weather patterns so that the planet maintains harmony.

This exercise can be found on **TRACK 10, DISC 2** of the included CDs.

There is a temple in Arcturus called Ra Mu Ma that is dedicated to the goddess within. It is important to connect with this goddess because she births new life. The feminine brings new energy and new life. We would like to take you on a journey to the Temple of Ra Mu Ma.

1. Close your eyes, and focus on your heart. Place your hand on your heart.

2. Gently breathe and be in silence. Breathe. You might hear the beat of your heart. The intention is that each beat takes you to your inner core. You go deeper and deeper into yourself.

3. Go to the place of the vesica piscis in your heart. Seek this place, and drink from the well of Mother/Father God.

4. When you feel nourished by the love of Mother/Father God, ask to be taken to the Temple of Ra Mu Ma. Visualize your personal merkabah — in any form or shape — appearing in front of you. Get into this merkabah. Your thoughts bring our energy, which takes you to that place.

5. Imagine that you are traveling to the Temple of Ra Mu Ma. This is a great temple shaped like a dome. When you arrive, you are led into a chamber, and there is a spinning ball of sacred fire.

6. Hold the globe of sacred fire with both hands. This globe spins gently in your hands. Breathe it in. Feel the energy from this globe go into your palms, activating the chakras there and flowing through your entire body. This energy settles in the middle of your forehead and your medulla oblongata.

7. Rest both hands above your ears so that your middle fingers touch the top of your head. Breathe it in. Breathe it in.

8. The Grand Goddess Ra Mu Ma comes and stands in front of you. She looks like a Mayan goddess. She has a feather in her hands. She touches your heart with her feather, sending electrical impulses into your body. You may bring your hands down now.

9. This electrical energy shines into your heart, your eyes, your third eye, and the middle of your forehead (your angel chakra), and it spreads into your brain, projecting a being behind you. This being is at least 15 feet tall. Breathe it in. Breathe it in. This being is your monad energy. Your monad is the energy of your soul group. Be with this energy.

10. You are standing, and the being behind you joins with you. This is you. Goddess Ra Mu Ma passes her feather through your heart, and it sends electrical energy through you to your monad.

11. A star appears atop your monad. The star shines and starts to spin. It sends light all over you. You integrate your monadic energy.

12. Goddess Ra Mu Ma touches your heart again with her feather, sending more energy. Visualize yourself expanding. You're getting taller and bigger. You are joining your monad. You have become 10 feet tall. Breathe it in.

13. You look at the shining star. It has become three stars, pouring light into you. Be in this space for a moment.

14. Goddess Ra Mu Ma now touches your forehead again with her feather, sending further electrical energy into your brain. This energy shoots upward, going all the way up to your twelfth and thirty-third chakras. Light beams up from your monad about 10 feet above you. Breathe it in.

15. Open your fingers now. The light from your thirty-third chakra streams out and spreads all around you. This is bright, liquid light coming from your hands. Feel the warmth of this light.

16. Cup your hands and bring them to your heart. Say, "I am the light."

I am the light.

17. "Every cell of my body is filled with this light."

Every cell of my body is filled with this light.

18. "I am becoming a beam of light."

I am becoming a beam of light.

19. "From now on, I am the monad. I am not a soul anymore. I am the monad. I am the group energy."

From now on, I am the monad. I am not a soul anymore. I am the group energy.

20. Breathe it in. You may bring your hand down now. Place your hands on your stomach, sending energy into your stomach.

21. See a beautiful merkabah appear with two pyramids joined, and say, "I anchor this energy in my solar plexus."

I anchor this energy in my solar plexus.

22. "This is my truth."

This is my truth.

23. You may bring your hands down now. Acknowledge the Goddess Ra Mu Ma. Thank her for the gifts she gave you.

I thank you for the gifts you gave me.

24. "In opening the higher part of myself today."

In opening the higher part of myself today.

25. Before she leaves, she gives you her white feather. She makes the white feather vibrate. Bring the white feather into your meditations, and use it to touch your heart and your forehead. You will activate energies with this feather. This is her gift to you.

Blessings. This is Archangel Metatron.

Thank you.

Family of God: You may open your eyes now.

Yes. Part of me is still there.

How do you feel, brother?

Very good. Part of me is still coming back from this. It is amazing.

It is better to stay there. This is an initiation.

Secrets of the Universe

Spectrum Light

Creator: When you see sunlight coming through a crystal, a prism, or a drop of water, you don't usually see many colors. You see a combination of colors, but two or three colors are predominant — hues of purple, white, and sometimes yellow, but you don't see all the colors. Think this through.

This spectrum of colors can be captured by a crystal from sunlight coming through a window. It can be captured and stored, and this stored energy can be used to change frequencies in the human body. It can be directed to parts of the body where there is a debilitating sickness. For example, this spectrum of light is very beneficial for people who have rheumatism, joint pain, and stiff necks, as well as for the overall well-being of the human body.

We encourage you to think about this: Can you capture this energy in an image? Hundreds — even thousands — of beings come together in a spectrum of light. They are called particle-of-light beings.

You can experiment. Take an unripe mango or another piece

of unripe fruit, and pass this spectrum of colors into the fruit. The fruit will ripen in a very short span of time. It will reach its maturity quickly. In the same way, human maturity is oneness. You can achieve oneness using the spectrum of light.

There are sensors on the back of your head. They are like invisible eyes, and they perceive this light spectrum. You are able to see vivid colors because of these sensors. When they are fully open and finely tuned, you will start appreciating the beauty that is all around you, from a little flower to a great landscape.

You can bring the spectrum of colors to your wallet or your money purse so that there will be harmony in your finances. Sixty percent of what most people carry in their wallets is junk — old scraps of paper or odds and ends from long ago. They do not understand that they are carrying dead energy in their wallets. How can they have money? Their wallets have not been replenished with the new energies. Bring the light spectrum into your wallet.

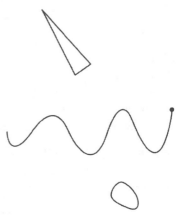

Figure 33.1. Light spectrum symbol to carry in your wallet

Here is the symbol for the light spectrum [figure 33.1]. It is good to carry this symbol in your wallet and also place it somewhere in your home.

Activate Codes on Your Fingertips

There are codes with chakras under your fingernails and on your fingertips. They transmit healing energies. When they are activated, you will be able to easily regulate the energies of receiving and giving. You will be able to receive easily and also share easily. There must be a flow. These images are for you to use to create flow in your life.

How do we activate these energy points in the fingers?

There is DNA under your fingernails. Focus on the area behind the fingernails and breathe. You will feel a coolness come into them. Can you feel the energy renewal?

Very much so. They're tingling very subtly, and it feels cool, which is unusual.

When these are activated, the energy in your life will flow in both directions — receiving and giving, giving and receiving. The flow will be much easier. But this is not about giving and receiving. It is about establishing a continuous flow of energy. It has nothing to do with the money. It has to do with energy flow. When you activate these chakras, simply close your eyes, ask Creator for help to activate them, and breathe into them.

Infinity-Sign Creation

In quiet moments, make infinity signs. Wherever you are comfortable sitting, make infinity signs with your index finger in the air. It is very simple. In 13 days, you will see more flow in your life. You will start to see more movement in your life. When there's movement, more energy flows.

Raindrops

There are many magical cures. People think of raindrops as just water falling. Yes, they are water falling, but there is much more to it. Each drop of rain contains the golden elixir of life. If you partake of rain — not rain containing chemical residue, but rain in its natural setting where it falls — and you stand beneath it, being bathed by falling rain, you will be able to balance your chakras and the elements within you. You can easily integrate many higher frequencies of energy by staying in falling rain.

The energy of Gaia is in raindrops. There is also the energy of Archangel Gabriel, Archangel Michael, and Mother Mary. Why do you think human beings like water? Water contains all these energies. Children play in water, splashing and happily laughing, feeling the energy of these masters.

Hold a drop of rain in your hand, and breathe into it. Your can have a transcendental experience and join again with All That Is. Rain is excellent medicine for curing many illnesses in the physical body. This is why in some shamanic traditions, shamans recommend taking a bath beneath a waterfall every day for a few days. The water flows in the forest on the rocks. It carries mineral components of the earth combined with components of the leaves and roots of the trees, and it can have a dramatic effect. It can strengthen your energetic field and immune system. It can heal many itches, pains, and scratches. The effects can be cleared and healed.

We wish to reveal this today. It might not make sense to some people. Some will say that this is impossible or absurd; nevertheless, we wish to bring this out. Every raindrop contains sound frequencies. People like to hear the sound of rain falling. One of your famous singers even wrote a song, "Raindrops Keep Falling on My Head." There is rhythm and melody in the rain, and it contains particles of gold.

When you partake of this beautiful gift, you open your heart more fully. Look at a photograph of a raindrop. You will see a spectrum of colors emanating from it. These beautiful colors represent the higher aspects of your chakras in higher realities.

You can make an intention and place it in raindrops. The rain is not just water. It is an essence. There is an intention behind it. There is coordination in it. There is love in it. It coordinates with the earth, the wind, and the clouds, determining how much water will fall, where it will rain, and whether the drops are large or small. There is a coherence of four forces coming together for rain.

A time will come when this is understood, and you will be able to coordinate these four aspects — the earth spirit, the wind spirit, the cloud spirit, and the rain spirit — to create things in life. You can do this by placing a drop of rain with your intention on your forehead, your third eye, and asking it to circulate throughout your body. Rain has the capacity to open your hearing to very high ranges so that you can hear the truth, smell the truth, and be the truth.

Your true nature is water. All of you are water beings. You are born from your mother's womb after the water breaks from your mother's uterus. This represents swimming in the ocean. Come back to the holy presence of water.

There is mathematics in each raindrop combined with geometric patterns. There is a symbol for rain with a mathematical number [see figure 33.2] Each raindrop contains this geometric pattern. Place this symbol in your house and in your wallet, and you will see the flow of energy in your life.

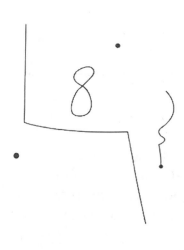

Figure 33.2. Symbol for rain

You must remember: Everything is spiritual energy, mathematics, and geometric codes. During the coming months, you will start to understand the decoding of the DNA. (We are preparing brother Rae for this.) There are sacred geometry patterns and musical frequencies combined with the mathematical equations inside DNA. With this simple diagram, you will experience energy flowing into your life.

Ask to Change Your Dense Thought Patterns

Commander Ashtar and King Akhenaton: Many truths and secrets are being revealed. It is said that when the student is ready, the teacher appears through perfect wisdom in embracing and seeking to experience the oneness. You create an energetic invitation. You open a door when you say, "I am ready to receive," and the energy of your intention is transmitted all the way to the Great Central Sun in a nanosecond, where the answers are downloaded.

When you seek higher truth, you must hold this intention constantly on an ongoing basis. This is how you experience more of the Divine. When you do not have the intention of seeking truth, your energy becomes stagnant. There is no growth.

Human beings fail to understand that they are part of the universe. You are part of the cosmos, and your thoughts and energies are picked up and read by the beings on the other side. Perhaps you are not aware that you can send your thought projections to the other side. There are legions of beings waiting to make an energetic connection. These legions are either of the light or the lower ones. Using sound and the spectrum of colors, you can pierce the veil, and your vibratory pattern of light will draw forth other patterns of light from the cosmos. That is why almost all higher frequency energy is thought.

We have machines in our spaceship that capture thought images, process them, refine them, and send them out again. Human beings have been producing heavy, dense thoughts. Now there are billions and billions of dense thoughts. They encircle Earth, and higher energies and higher light cannot pierce the density. We have been refining this energy, but the volume is increasing exponentially. Human beings are creating more dense patterns of thought.

Individually, you can ask us to refine your thoughts. We invite you to come to our ship and ask, "How can I change my thought patterns from dense thoughts to lighter thoughts?" We will connect our machines to your brain and your body, and we will remove many dense thought-energy creators, which are experiences of the past that create dense energies that continuously replay. When these experiences are removed, the process of creating dense thoughts is lessened.

We also have machines that reflect higher-vibrational thought back into your body, changing your vibratory pattern and cellular structure. These recode (not decode) you to your original light. You will be able to return to your highest light. But you must ask for this.

We are bringing you this information for the first time. Good day to all of you. This is King Akhenaton and Commander Ashtar.

Harmonize Your Life

Maha Avatar Babaji: "I exist in each grain of sand." I am sure you have heard this saying. It means each grain of sand contains the consciousness of All That Is. And how is a grain of sand created? It didn't fall from the sky. It was created using sound combined with the color spectrum. When you use sound with the color spectrum, the spectrum of colors is crushed, and small particles of light fall all over.

Sound can be used to create a light spectrum to crush things to various sizes — big, small, medium, any size you want. Every act of creation comes from sound.

You can fine-tune sounds to create anything, and there is a sound frequency attached to everything. Discover the sound of the mountain, the sound of the forest, the sound of the earth, the sound of a cloud, or the sound of water. When you combine these, you harmonize with creation and Earth, and when you are in harmony with creation, your music sounds very good in the orchestra of life. You become one with the flow.

Most people are not able to create because they are not in the flow. Everything has to be harmonized. This simply means cognizing with the primordial consciousness. "Cognize" means understand.

The secrets of the universe are for people who are ready to work with them, people who work with shifted energy. This happened because of the new vibration and because of the shift that happened.

There are microscopic lines on an apple. What do they mean? These lines carry electromagnetic frequency. They are directly related to the frequencies of Mother Earth. They are connected to the grid lines. When you connect with the grid, you are in harmony with every aspect of your life. Everything in your life comes from Earth. When you touch an apple, you are holding Earth in your hand. Understand what an apple is.

Gaia: When you are holding an apple, you are holding me in your hands. When you hold any food, you are holding me, for my energy is in everything that grows on me. The grid lines on an apple reflect the twelve main grid lines on my body, and everything that is created on me contains these important grid lines:

1. Michael line (blue)
2. Guanyin line (soft blue)
3. Melchizedek line (platinum)
4. Mother Mary line (soft pink)
5. St. Germain and Lady Portia line (violet)
6. Maitreya line (soft green)
7. Sophia line (soft white)
8. Unicorn line (white)
9. Devayani line (gold)
10. Commander Ashtar line (soft blue)
11. Thoth line (orange)
12. Dragon line (metallic green)

These twelve grid lines exist on everything and everyone that is created on my body.

Afterword
Achieve Understanding to Change Your Perspective

The Celestial Beings

We are the celestial beings. We all are here — Mahareya, Akhenaton, Michael, and all who have supported this project. We come forward to say thank you for your dedication to using the methods we provided and for taking the time to bring this understanding of ascension about in this new way.

This book is a light for those who seek their higher selves. It is a light for those who are already on spiritual paths whose accomplishments are rapidly advancing as they use the techniques presented here.

After reading it, those with just a cursory interest in understanding ascension will have gained more than they expected. When you read a few lines or a few words and visualize the images, this creates thought patterns that generate energy that you will continue to experience in the coming years. You will see the deeper meanings behind these written words.

If you reread this material in three years, you will acquire even deeper levels of understanding from the energy behind the words.

We encourage you to work with the tools given here, even if just for short periods, and you will learn how to shift your perceptions.

Your ascension is simply a change in how you look at life. It is how you are able to see through the eyes of truth, how you are able to see and experience the oneness. Working through the methods in this book provides answers for that.

Congratulations, Graduate!

We welcome you into this new you. It is a new version of you in the status of a graduate — not from college but rather with a double PhD in the deeper aspects of life. You are the light of the world. We are with you always.

We are the Celestial Beings — Akhenaton, Mahareya, Michael, and others. We bless you and hold you in the divine love of the Creator.

ABOUT

ℛae Chandran

Rae Chandran was born in India and has lived in the United States and Japan. He performs individual channeling sessions for his clients, and his articles have been published in the *Sedona Journal of Emergence.* Rae teaches workshops throughout the Far East on the Ancient Egyptian mysteries, DNA activation, and channeling. He creates soul 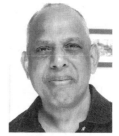 symbols for his clients, and he leads tours of ancient holy places worldwide.

Rae founded the Omran Institute, which promotes DNA awareness and certifies practitioners of Omran 12-Strand DNA Activation. He also performs individual Omran 12-Strand DNA sessions for his clients. Rae lives with his wife and children outside of Tokyo, Japan. For more information, visit his website at RaeChandran.com.

Robert Mason Pollock

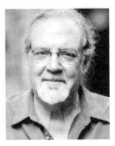

Robert Mason Pollock was born in Washington, DC, and has lived in London (England), Canada, and the Berkshire mountains of Massachusetts. He is an energy healer at a holistic health resort in the Berkshires, and he has an energy healing practice with locations in New York City and the Berkshires.

Robert wrote *Navigating by Heart*. He teaches workshops in spirituality and DNA activation. He also performs individual Omran 12-Strand DNA sessions for his clients. For more information, visit his website at BerkshireEnergyHealing.com.

Light Technology PUBLISHING Presents

TO ORDER PRINT BOOKS
Visit LightTechnology.com, Call 928-526-1345 or 1-800-450-0985,
or Check Amazon.com or Your Favorite Bookstore

THROUGH RAE CHANDRAN WITH ROBERT MASON POLLOCK

Angels and Ascension: Integrate Celestial Energy for a Benevolent Life

Includes Mudras, Breathing Exercises, and Intonations!

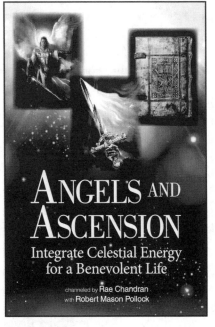

Much support is available for humanity. Angelic support has always been available, but people did not know about it because they were looking for a tangible support system — something they could see, feel, or touch. In the new consciousness, you must learn to believe in the unseen. Know support is available if you focus.

The angels completely support every human soul on the planet as well as all animals, plants, and trees, but you must ask for this support system to be activated. We bring the understanding of angels so that you can work with them to find joy, peace, and freedom in your heart. We encourage you to speak with all your friends and family about the benefits of working with angels. Work with angels every day, and you will see the difference.

Chapters Include
- Enhance Your Senses and Vitality
- Boost Your Mental Facilities
- Expand Your Consciousness
- Use Numbers to Improve Your Life
- Principles for Examining Doctrine to Make Sound Decisions
- Find Your Blueprint and Life Plan
- Clear Karmic Energy
- Spiritual Cosmology
- Ascension Practices
- Angelic Energy Practices
- Mudras for Angelic Support

$16.95 • Softcover • 6 x 9 • 176 PP.
ISBN 978-1-62233-048-5

THROUGH RAE CHANDRAN WITH ROBERT MASON POLLOCK

Dance of the Hands

Dance of the Hands is for everyone, not just people who are spiritually advanced. It is for any layperson, regardless of religion. This material is for those who have an interest in bettering themselves or improving their well-being — practitioners, teachers, masters, the spiritually advanced, neophytes, and children.

The purpose of these mudras is to balance the body, mind, and soul. Like any spiritual practice, doing mudras brings balance to every area of your life. The benefits are simple as well: These mudras bring joy and peace to your life. When you are joyful and peaceful, you are more likely to access the higher aspects of your consciousness.

Practicing these mudras can bring you a sense of calmness, well-being, and heightened awareness. Each person will have individual results. Over time, you will notice a sense of balance and empowerment coming into your life. Relationships can be healed and reconciled. You will become more tolerant, more accepting, and less judgmental.

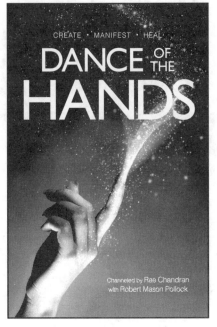

CREATE • MANIFEST • HEAL

DANCE OF THE HANDS

Channeled by Rae Chandran with Robert Mason Pollock

Learn mudras that help you
- unify the body, mind, and soul
- connect with the elements
- express with heartfelt communication
- boost energy to complete a task
- balance between male and female polarities
- calm anxiety and fear
- relieve challenging energy in your daily life
- protect your energy field
- create healthy eating habits
- feel safe and secure in your environment
- bring back lost parts of your consciousness

$16.95 • Softcover • 6 x 9 • 160 PP.
ISBN 978-1-62233-038-6
Lay flat book with wire-o binding

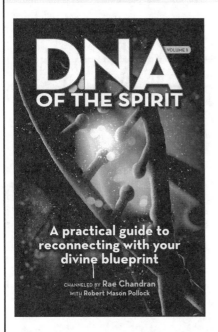
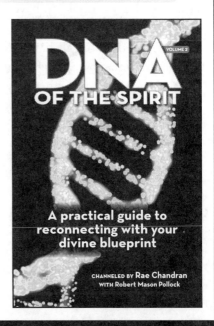

THROUGH RAE CHANDRAN WITH ROBERT MASON POLLOCK

Partner with Angels and Benefit Every Area of Your Life

Angels are the Creator's workforce, and in this book, individual angels describe their responsibilities and explain how they can help you with all aspects of your life — practical and spiritual. All you need to do is ask.

The purpose of this material is to bring the awareness of angels in a much more practical, easy-to-understand way. Call on the angels to show you the potential you have in your life to create a new reality.

Many of these angels have never spoken to human beings before or revealed their names or what they do. Here are some examples of what you will find inside:

- **La Banaha**, the essence of the Moon, explains feminine empowerment and organ rejuvenation.
- **Angel Anauel** describes fair commerce.
- **Angel Tahariel** helps you purify and shift your vibration.
- **Angel Mansu** gives advice about how to eliminate the trauma from birthing procedures.
- **Angel Agon** inspires writers and filmmakers and relates how you can call on him for inspiration.

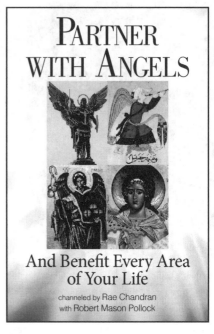

PARTNER WITH ANGELS

And Benefit Every Area of Your Life

channeled by Rae Chandran
with Robert Mason Pollock

- **Angel Tadzekiel** helps you access your wisdom and put it into perspective.
- **Archangel Maroni** downloads your individual pathway to ascension.

Chapters Include
- The Benefits of Working with Angels
- Prepare for a New Consciousness
- Design Your Unique Path
- Access Support from Celestial Bodies
- Invoke Vibrational Support and Activation
- Practice Universal Communication
- Develop Environmental Connections
- You Are the New Masters

$16.95 • Softcover • 6 x 9 • 208 PP.
ISBN 978-1-62233-034-8

⚜ 𝓛𝓲𝓰𝓱𝓽 𝓣𝓮𝓬𝓱𝓷𝓸𝓵𝓸𝓰𝔂 PUBLISHING Presents

TO ORDER PRINT BOOKS
Visit LightTechnology.com, Call 928-526-1345 or 1-800-450-0985,
or Check Amazon.com or Your Favorite Bookstore

THROUGH RAE CHANDRAN

Rumi's Songs of the Soul

Artwork by Yizhao Zhang

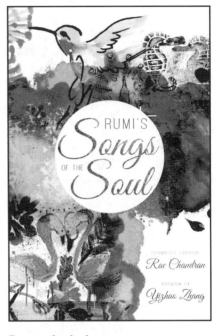

What is not known about me is that I was greatly influenced by the understandings and philosophy of the magi who were the followers of the sacred fire. I had thoughts put into my mind while I slept and during times of deep silence about the sacredness of all life and about how to accept things in life without discarding any of it. I followed this and never gave up on finding God, for in rejecting any part of God, I was rejecting God entirely.

Now in modern times, people must carefully examine what supported them before and make adjustments and corrections wherever necessary. I wanted to bring my writings in a newer form that would suit your present Earth reality because of the changing times and planetary shift. To do this, I chose my old student, Rae (he was one of the students at the seminary in Konya), to bring forth this new understanding to help people remember the Law of One and the Family of God.

I offer these poems in humble gratitude.

— Rumi

Poems Include

- The Celestial Home
- Challenges and Difficulties
- Divine Lovers
- Tribute to Mothers
- The Love You Seek
- Silence and Solitude
- The Night Sky
- Enlightenment
- The Beauty of Animals
- Self-Realization
- The Soul of Love

$15.95 • Softcover • 6 x 9 • 128 PP.
ISBN 978-1-62233-059-1

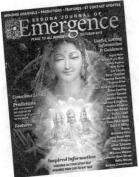
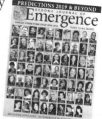

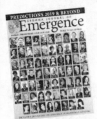
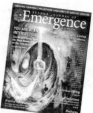

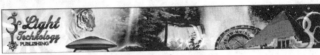
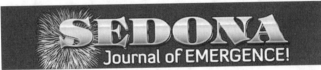

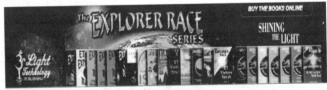

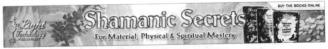